EVIDENCE-BASED PATIENT HANDLING

Providing care and treatment for patients usually requires moving and handling activities associated with high rates of back injury in health and social-care staff. Over the last twenty years a number of guidelines have been published, based on professional consensus, but to date there has been no appraisal of the research evidence. This book reports a systematic review which fills that gap and tackles the challenge of producing an evidence base to support clinical practice.

Evidence-based Patient Handling looks at the evidence relating to:

- controversial techniques
- patient-handling tasks
- equipment used in these tasks
- interventions used to reduce injuries.

The tasks section includes summary flow charts of the current guidelines for seven key tasks, for example transferring from sitting-to-sitting and care and repositioning in lying. These options are then discussed in terms of the different levels of supporting evidence. The interventions section looks at programmes aimed at reducing injuries, including initiatives based on risk assessment, training, ergonomics and lifting teams. The findings challenge previously-held opinions about moving and handling and provide the foundation for future practice.

Evidence-based Patient Handling breaks new ground in a fundamental area of day-to-day work in health and social care. It provides a wide range of professionals with a much-needed source of reference, including: nurses, back-care advisors, health-care managers, risk managers, physiotherapists, occupational therapists, midwives, ergonomists, occupational health practitioners (including doctors), ambulance services, and health-staff educators.

Sue Hignett is a Lecturer in Ergonomics at Loughborough University. **Emma Crumpton** is a Consultant Ergonomist. **Sue Ruszala** is a Manual Handling and Ergonomics Advisor, United Bristol Healthcare NHS Trust. **Pat Alexander** is a Consultant Back Care Advisor. **Mike Fray** is a self-employed Ergonomics and Rehabilitation Advisor. **Brian Fletcher** is a Freelance Consultant.

EVIDENCE-BASED PATIENT HANDLING

Tasks, Equipment and Interventions

Sue Hignett, Emma Crumpton, Sue Ruszala,
Pat Alexander, Mike Fray and Brian Fletcher

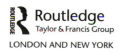
Routledge
Taylor & Francis Group

LONDON AND NEW YORK

First published 2003
by Routledge
11 New Fetter Lane, London EC4P 4EE

Simultaneously published in the USA and Canada
by Routledge
29 West 35th Street, New York, NY 10001

Routledge is an imprint of the Taylor & Francis Group

© 2003 Sue Hignett, Emma Crumpton, Sue Ruszala,
Pat Alexander, Mike Fray, Brian Fletcher

Typeset in Sabon by Bookcraft Ltd, Stroud, Gloucestershire
Printed and bound in Great Britain by TJ International Ltd,
Padstow, Cornwall

British Library Cataloguing in Publication Data
A catalogue record for this book is available from the British Library

Library of Congress Cataloging in Publication Data
Evidence-based patient handling: tasks, equipment, and interventions/
Sue Hignett ... [et al].
p. cm.
Includes bibliographical references and index.
1. Evidence-based medicine. 2. Medical personnel and patient.
3. Continuum of care. 4. Medical care.
I. Hignett, Sue (Susan), 1960–
RC48 .E954 2002
616–dc21   2002068227

ISBN 0–415–24631–8 (hbk)
ISBN 0–415–24632–6 (pbk)

CONTENTS

ILLUSTRATIONS

FIGURES

TABLES

ACKNOWLEDGEMENTS

All the project team would like to thank their partners and families for their support over the two years it has taken for this book to come to fruition. In particular we are grateful to Emma and Joe's baby for not being born until the manuscript was complete!

The project team support was excellent and we would like to acknowledge the contributions of the following: Michael Dewey (Deputy Director of Trent Institute for Health Services Research, University of Nottingham), Julie Glanville (Associate Director, NHS Centre for Reviews and Dissemination of Information, University of York), Rob Goodwin (search and administration), Laura Norton (flow charts), Margery Swift (administration), John Rule, Priscilla and Ann at Nottingham City Hospital (search and library services), Lynn Clarke and Tony Norcross (translations).

We are extremely grateful for the financial support from the Health and Safety Executive (RSU ref. 4160/R55.092) and the NHS Executive (Trent) (ref. RBG 01XX3). Without this support the level of detail achieved in the project would not have been possible.

PART I

RESEARCH BACKGROUND
AND CRITERIA

CHAPTER 1

INTRODUCTION AND BACKGROUND

Patient-handling activities, as primary or secondary tasks, are carried out by health-care staff (and other carers) in all professional groups throughout the health-care industry. Since 1992 there has been specific legislation on manual handling (MHOR, 1992) which has been driving forward the initiative to reduce musculoskeletal injuries in the health-care industry. Over the last twenty years a number of guidance publications have been published, some conflicting and some controversial. These have been used operationally throughout the health-care industry to guide clinical practice and, additionally, as reference texts for expert opinion in legal proceedings. To date there has been no substantial text that places the advice about patient-handling techniques and equipment in the context of published research rather than as expert opinion or anecdotes.

The six authors had all worked and researched in the field of patient handling for many years and felt that, with the increasing emphasis on clinical governance and the growing culture of litigation in the UK for patient-handling-related injuries, clinical tasks which included patient handling should be evidenced-based as far as possible.

The aim of this book is to bring together all available research in a systematic literature review framework with the hope of providing a foundation for future guidance publications. It is divided into two parts:

Part I sets out the background to the research and the research criteria.

Part II details the results from the literature examined during the research. This part is set out in four sections to look at the literature pertaining to:

- controversial techniques and hazardous tasks (Chapter 3);
- patient-handling tasks – including specialist areas (Chapters 4, 5 and 6);
- equipment used in these tasks (Chapters 7, 8 and 9); and
- interventions to reduce injuries associated with patient handling (Chapters 10 and 11).

The chapters are further divided into subsections to group the relevant literature. Each subsection begins with an introduction which summarises the analysis of the included literature. At the end of each subsection is a box giving the statements of the evidence levels with the quality rating (QR) and practitioner rating (PR). There is a glossary at the end of the book giving additional information on some of the measurement tools and abbreviations.

1.1   RESEARCH QUESTIONS

Before we could get started we had to set out our research questions so that we could return to them at the end of the project to see what, if anything, had been achieved.

1   Can research be found on the techniques and equipment recommended by current guidance publications for specific patient-handling tasks?
2   What are the results from the research?
3   How do these results compare with the current guidance available?
4   How do individual techniques and equipment compare with other techniques/ equipment for the same task?

Although we have been working in the area of manual handling for patients for a number of years we still find that we get caught up in popular notions for practice rather than asking if they are evidence-based. For this reason the following publications were reviewed: Disabled Living Foundation (2001); Essex Group of National Back Exchange (1996); The Disability Information Trust (1996); Royal College of Midwives (1997); Lloyd *et al.* (National Back Pain Association/Royal College of Nursing, 1998, revised edition); South London and Kent Group, National Back Exchange (1998); Health Services Advisory Committee (1998); Chartered Society of Physiotherapy (1998); Oxford Region, National Back Exchange (1999); ASSTSAS (1999); Human Services/Victorian Work cover Authority (1999); Graham *et al.* (2000); The Resuscitation Council (2001); Derbyshire Interagency Group (2001). These publications were used to develop the flow charts at the start of the sections in Chapters 4 and 5.

   We have included a summary of different options for carrying out each task (Chapters 4 and 5) and, where possible, have given an indication of the evidence supporting the options. Each flow chart has three action boxes:

1   Hands Off: by supervision and verbal prompts and/or providing equipment to facilitate completely independent movement by the patient;
2   Hands On (some help): giving assistance using manual techniques and/or equipment with the patient assisting the movement, transfer, care or repositioning task;
3   Hands On (a lot of help): moving dependent patients who are assessed as mostly unable or unsuitable to give assistance (e.g. non-weight-bearing and/or uncooperative).

Many of the recommended techniques from the professional guidance publications are not referred to in the evidence literature. This means that no evidence was found from this search to suggest whether these techniques are appropriate or not for either patients or carers. Where possible descriptions of techniques and equipment have been included in the extract, but you may also find it helpful, for clarity and more detail, to look at the original paper and/or contact the authors of the original papers.

Chapter 2 sets out the methodology used for the review. It contains information about the search strategy, inter-rater reliability, extraction/appraisal form used and data synthesis. We decided to include all study types rather than only seeking what some consider the highest forms of evidence (meta-analyses, systematic reviews and randomised controlled trials). There were two reasons for this inclusive decision:

1   we thought that there might not be any papers at the highest forms of evidence; and
2   philosophically there is debate about the logic for claiming a high status for quantitative-based studies when issues of realism, external validity and social factors are considered (Murphy *et al.*, 1998).

Chapter 3 reviews controversial techniques. A decision was made to include Troup *et al.* (1981), Lloyd *et al.* (1987), Corlett *et al.* (1992), Lloyd *et al.* (1998, revised), ASSTSAS (1999) and Derbyshire Interagency Group (2001). The first four give an overview of the recommendations from the Royal College of Nursing (UK) over the last twenty years, together with a view from Canada (ASSTSAS, 1999) and a more recent consensus document from Derbyshire (UK). We apologise if we have missed learned publications from other countries and would be most interested in seeing other professional guidelines.

1.2   SUMMARY OF FINDINGS

Over 2,790 document titles were retrieved. We read, appraised and extracted data from over 880 papers and retained over 225 papers as extracts.

The results from the research are summarised in each of the sections and, although we have not always compared the findings with the recommendations in current guidance, there are several key points as shown in Table 1 which will, we are sure, be discussed with interest.

Only one section (10.1) produced a strong-evidence-level statement with four studies with a QR ≥75 per cent. This evidence statement that training interventions predominantly based on training/education have no impact on working practices or injury rates is further backed up by the lack of strong evidence for Section 10.3 (positive outcomes). It is now time for the health care industry, especially nurses as the largest professional group, to take stock and look at the alternatives to training for managing the back-pain problem. Chapter 11 gives indications of the type of interventions which should be considered, ranging from single-factor through to multi-factor interventions (with a range of different factors). All the options have a moderate-evidence level, although Section 11.1 (interventions based on risk assessment) has the most research, with nineteen papers.

Table 1 Summary of evidence: strong and moderate levels

Section	Task, equipment, intervention	Evidence level	Number of studies
3.2	Shoulder lift presents less risk than the orthodox lift, through-arm lift, under-arm drag and barrow lift	moderate	3
3.4	Hazardous tasks involve moving patients in bed; bed–chair transfers; toileting; bathing; and lifting from the floor	moderate	7
4.2.1	Use mechanical hoists to transfer from sitting for dependent (non-weight-bearing) patients	moderate	3
4.2.1 7.3	Use a walking belt with two carers to transfer from sitting for weight-bearing patients	moderate	5
4.2.1 7.3	Do not use a walking belt with one carer to transfer from sitting for weight-bearing patients	moderate	3
4.2.1	A belt lifter (standing hoist) may be preferable to manual techniques to transfer from sitting	moderate	2
5.1.1	Use a piqué (waterproof padded sheet, similar to a drawsheet) for turning a patient in bed	moderate	2
6.1.1	Ambulance work can result in harmful postures, with the highest risks involving the transportation of patients on equipment	moderate	3
6.4.1	Manual-handling difficulties for community nursing are associated with patient beds	moderate	3
6.4.3	Using multi-factor interventions, based on risk assessment, for community problems reduces lost time due to back pain	moderate	3
8.1	Support for the use of adjustable-height beds for caring tasks	moderate	3
8.2	Electric beds reduce the physical strain relating to nursing/manual-handling tasks associated with caring for patients in bed	moderate	2
9.1	There are complex reasons for why hoists are not used to their full capacity. These include staff attitude, lack of training, lack of availability, lack of knowledge, difficulties in attaching slings and lack of space	moderate	4
9.2	Hoist design (overhead and mobile) could be improved	moderate	2
9.3	Sling use and comfort are compromised by difficulties in selecting the correct size, the design of the leg pieces, and the method of application	moderate	2

10.1	Training interventions have no impact on working practices or injury rates	strong	4 (strong) 8 (mod)
10.2	Training interventions can have mixed short- term results	moderate	2
10.3	Training interventions can have positive short-term outcomes	moderate	4
11.1	Interventions based on risk assessments show improvements in measurement criteria	moderate	10
11.1	Managers and supervisors tend to support training/education interventions whereas workers (staff) support the provision of physical aids (equipment)	moderate	2
11.2	Moderate evidence from three studies that multi-factor interventions can show improvements. Contradictory evidence from one high-quality study which showed no improvement from a multi-factor intervention	moderate	3
11.3	Single-factor interventions based on the provision of equipment can be effective	moderate	2
11.4	Interventions using the lifting-team approach are effective	moderate	3

When considering the comparison of individual techniques and equipment with other techniques/equipment for the same task, Chapters 3, 4 and 5 raise some interesting questions. The controversial techniques need revisiting as some of the decisions to change practice, or condemn techniques, do not seem to have been evidence-based. The use of a walking belt (around the patient) with two carers has moderate evidence from five studies, whereas the use of the walking belt with one carer should be discouraged. The role for mechanical hoists seems to be limited to dependent patients who are not weight bearing, with the reasons for why hoists are not used (Section 9.1) perhaps contributing to this limitation.

Height-adjustable (especially electric) beds have a moderate-evidence level for reducing physical strain, although there is perhaps room for more research in this area. We have found a range of research addressing most areas of patient handling, although mostly with only two or three papers supporting the moderate-evidence statement levels. Notable omissions include paediatric handling, assisting patients in walking, emergency handling (e.g. resuscitation, fire evacuation) and rehabilitation (treatment handling).

We hope that all health-care staff who are involved in patient handling will find this information useful. The next stage is to challenge the professional bodies and researchers to produce more evidence on which to base the clinical practices involving patient handling.

CHAPTER 2

METHOD OF SYSTEMATIC REVIEW

Since the early 1980s the health-care industry has used formal methods of systematically reviewing studies to produce reliable, useful summaries of the effects of health-care interventions. This type of information is then used to formulate guidelines and clinical strategies (Ukoumunne *et al.*, 1999; Cameron *et al.*, 2000). The development of this approach has been driven by both external (political) and internal (professional) pressures to base clinical decisions on scientific evidence.

Chalmers and Altman (1995) identified a number of applications for systematic reviews, with the most important being the ability to give an accurate assessment of the literature. They suggested that traditional (narrative) reviews could be criticised as being haphazard and biased by the individual reviewer; a more systematic approach would achieve greater reliability by allowing an assessment of how the review was carried out. Additional benefits include a more explicit definition of exclusion/inclusion criteria and the critical appraisal process and the possibility of explaining inconsistencies or conflicts in data which might relate to the sampling strategy or outcome measures, etc.

2.1 METHOD

Hamer and Collinson (1999) described the key components of a systematic review as being:

1 Definition of the research question (Chapter 1)
2 Methods for identifying the research studies (search strategy)
3 Selection of studies for inclusion
4 Quality appraisal of included studies
5 Extraction of the data
6 Synthesis of the data.

2.2   RESEARCH QUESTIONS

These were outlined in Chapter 1 as follows:

1   Can research be found on the techniques and equipment recommended by current guidance publications for specific patient-handling tasks?
2   What are the results from the research?
3   How do these results compare with the current guidance available?
4   How do individual techniques and equipment compare with other techniques/ equipment for the same task?

2.3   SEARCH

A search strategy (see example in Appendix 1) was developed with considerable advice from Dr Julie Glanville (Associate Director, NHS Centre for Reviews and Dissemination of Information, University of York) and Dr John Rule (Post-Graduate Library, Nottingham City Hospital NHS Trust).

The search was extended to include all languages and included a number of strategies (Hart, 1998; Hamer and Collinson, 1999) as shown in Table 2.

2.3.1   Translations

All languages were included in the search – where possible English extracts were obtained – with translation being arranged as required. Studies with no English extract had the extract translated for inclusion/exclusion screening before a decision for full translation was made.

Table 2 Search strategies and results

Source	Retrieved
Medline (1960–2001)	1130
AMED	34
Psychinfo	73
EMBASE	631
CINAHL	493
Ergonomics extracts	27
British nursing index	12
Best evidence	2
Hand searching journals and exploding the reference list of identified papers	47
Contacting expert informants and theses' authors	42
Personal collections	305
Total	2796

Thirty papers were translated from eleven languages: Chinese, Danish, Dutch, French, German, Italian, Japanese, Norwegian, Portuguese, Slovak, and Spanish.

2.4   INCLUSION/EXCLUSION CRITERIA

The next stage resulted in the elimination of duplications (from the different search strategies) and papers which were inappropriate to the research topic based on their title. The remaining 880 papers were included and sent to the project team for review. Subsequent eliminations were based on the following inclusion/exclusion criteria whereby a paper or document was:

1   included if it described a named task, piece(s) of equipment or intervention relating directly to patient handling;
2   included as a professional opinion if it had:

   - references,
   - critically appraised the literature,
   - provided a new interpretation of the literature;

3   excluded if it was related to epidemiology of musculoskeletal disorders (usually low-back pain) and did not meet Criterion 1 for the study;
4   excluded if it was not the primary source of a study. The primary source was sought and included;
5   excluded if it was a legal case law report.

2.5   APPRAISAL/EXTRACTION TOOL

All the project team had specialist experience in the area of patient handling and were concerned that there might be limited research which met the highest traditional criteria for systematic reviews (randomised controlled trials). Advice was sought from Dr Michael Dewey (MD), Deputy Director of Trent Institute for Health Services Research.

An appropriate checklist, which included both randomised and non-randomised studies, was identified (Downs and Black, 1998) and recommended for this project by MD. The Downs and Black (1998) checklist was used for all studies 'with an intervention'. In order to include a range of study types the checklist was modified for 'studies with no intervention' (see Figure 1 opposite) and 'other' types of studies. The modifications were tested within the project group before undergoing the inter-rater reliability trial. In order to include qualitative studies a checklist was developed (Grbich, 1999; Whalley-Hammell et al., 2000; Seale, 1999). A full copy of the data appraisal/extraction tool and score sheet can be found in appendix 2. Figure 1 and Table 3 show the decision-making hierarchy used in the appraisal/extraction process.

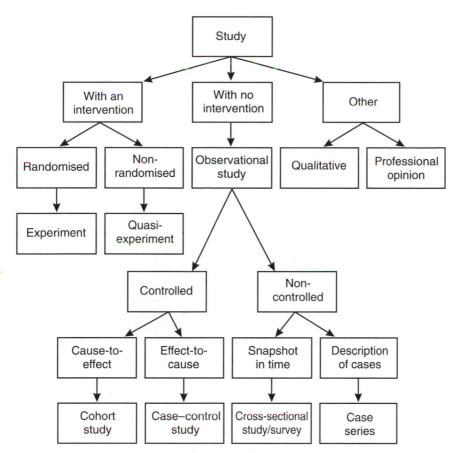

Figure 1 Design hierarchy for study type

The data appraisal/extraction tool produced scores in four sections with a final quality score. The four sections were:

1   reporting: assessing whether the information presented in the paper would allow the reader to make an unbiased assessment of the findings of the study;
2   external validity: assessing the extent that the findings from the study could be generalised to the population from which the study subject came;
3   bias: assessing the biases in the measurement of the intervention and outcome;
4   confounding: assessing the bias in the selection of the study subjects.

An additional reality check was added in the form of a five-point subjective Practitioner Rating score (Hignett's Convincing Scale, see Appendix 2 on page 188). This asked the reviewer to consider whether they would be likely to use the findings from the study in their practice regardless of the scientific quality of the paper.

Table 3 Study-type definitions

Study type	Definition	Abbreviation
Intervention – randomised	Concealed random allocation or pseudo-random allocation (e.g. alternate allocation or by birth date, etc.). Experimental design where a variable is manipulated and compared to a group where that variable was not manipulated.	expt
Intervention – non-randomised, quasi-experimental	Similar to true experiment. Has subjects, intervention, etc. but uses non-randomised groups.	quasi
Observational – controlled, cohort	Begin by identifying individuals with (study group) and without (control group) a factor being investigated. Observed over time. The actual observation may be retrospective or prospective. From cause to effect.	cohort
Observational – controlled case–control study	Usually retrospective study that begins by identifying individuals with common factors (cases) for comparison without the factor (controls). Analysis proceeds from effect to cause.	CCS
Observational – no control, cross-sectional study or survey	Descriptive study of the relationships between the outcome and population usually at one point in time, or one defined 'snapshot' period of time.	x-sect.
Observational – no control, case series	A clearly-identified group illustrating a point are defined and observed for a defined period of time. The cases are described; there is no control/comparison group.	case
Qualitative	Research involving the collection, analysis and interpretation of data which are not easily reduced to numbers.	qual.
Professional opinion	Individual opinion and/or group consensus based on experience rather than research.	PO

2.5.1   Inter-rater reliability

As the review process used two members of the project team to appraise and extract data from each paper, before the main part of the review commenced it was important to assess the inter-rater reliability of the reviewers. Ten papers were randomly selected and copies of each were sent to the members of the project team.

Inter-rater reliability was calculated using intraclass correlation coefficients (ICC). From this calculation of single-measure intraclass correlation, the ICC for two judges was calculated using the Spearman-Brown prophecy formula (Shrout and Fleiss, 1979). There was complete agreement, by all reviewers, on the study design type as shown in Table 4.

Table 4   Results of study design type

Study identification	Study design type
1 Charney et al., 1991	Quasi-experimental
2 Coleman, 1999	Cross-sectional study
3 Dehlin and Lindberg, 1975	Cross-sectional study
4 Ellis, 1993	Survey
5 Engels et al., 1994	Cross-sectional study
6 Fenety and Kumar, 1992	Survey
7 Finsen et al., 1998	Cross-sectional study
8 Fragala, 1993	Quasi-experimental
9 French et al., 1997	Cross-sectional study
10 Garg and Owen, 1991	Quasi-experimental

The results of the inter-rater reliability are shown in Table 5.

Table 5   Results of inter-rater reliability

Component	Pair-wise, intra-class correlation ($r =$)
Reporting	0.87
External validity	0.53
Bias	0.72
Confounding	0.76
Overall quality score	0.95

The individual components of the appraisal/extraction tool reliability varied from poor/moderate (external validity) to good (reporting, bias and confounding). The overall quality score showed good reliability ($r = 0.95$).

Downs and Black (1998) found similar results, with poor reliability for external validity (Spearman correlation coefficient $= -0.14$). They suggested that this might either be due to the small number of items in this section (three questions compared with six to ten in the other sections) or to the construction of the questions. The overall quality score showed good reliability ($r = 0.95$), which compared well with the findings of Downs and Black (1998), correlation $= 0.75$.

Inter-rater reliability was established, giving a level of confidence to the main review process.

2.6   DATA EXTRACTION

Each of the 880 papers/documents/theses were sent to two reviewers. Reviewers were not sent their own publications to review. The maximum permissible difference in the QR score was set at three by MD. Any difference greater than this was sent for conflict resolution to a third reviewer. The QR scores were then averaged to give the final scores shown in the 'Summary of evidence' tables at the end of each section.

Owing to the heterogeneity of the study types, interventions, settings, participants, outcome measures and comparison groups a quantitative analysis (meta-analysis) was not appropriate.

2.7   DATA SYNTHESIS

The data were synthesised in two stages. The first stage involved grouping papers into the categories of task, equipment or intervention with some papers being allocated to more than one category, so extracts may appear in more than one chapter to ensure that the individual sections contain all the relevant data to support the evidence statements. This was followed by agreeing evidence levels (Table 6) based on the QR scores from extraction/appraisal process. This table was developed from the evidence-level tables published by Bernard (1997) and the Faculty of Occupational Medicine (2000).

2.7.1   No evidence

It is important to note that a poor- or no-evidence level (☹) is not the same as negative evidence. For example in Chapter 10, there are three sections: the first presents the evidence which indicates that training, as the main component of an intervention, did not work; the second, the papers with mixed results; and the third, the papers which found that training had positive outcomes.

Most sections are not divided in this way. If no evidence is presented to give positive and negative findings it may just mean that this particular research question has not been investigated, rather than that a conclusion should be drawn about a particular task, a piece of equipment or an intervention strategy.

Table 6 Evidence levels	
☺☺☺☺	Strong evidence – provided by multiple (three or more), high-quality (QR ≥75% score) studies.
☺☺☺	Moderate evidence – provided by generally consistent findings in fewer (two or more), smaller or lower-quality (QR = 50–74% score) studies.
☺☺	Limited or contradictory evidence – provided one study (QR ≥50%), or findings in multiple (two or more) lower-quality (QR = 25–49% score) studies.
☹	Poor or no evidence – no studies or low-quality score (QR ≤24%).
(Bernard, 1997; Faculty of Occupational Medicine, 2000)	

2.7.2   Summary of evidence

The authors' terminology has been used as far as possible in the paper extracts. This was to avoid any interpretation by the project group which might have introduced bias. The extracts, therefore, are not an interpretation by, or the opinion of, the project group.

The interpretation by the project group is via:

1   the extraction and appraisal process; and
2   the evidence statements.

At each stage multiple reviewers have been used to minimise bias.

PART II

RESEARCH RESULTS

SECTION I

CONTROVERSIAL TECHNIQUES AND HAZARDOUS TASKS

CHAPTER 3

CONTROVERSIAL ISSUES

For many years certain techniques have been proscribed by various authoritative sources, for example professional bodies such as the Royal College of Nursing (UK) and Chartered Society of Physiotherapy (UK). Some, such as the drag lift, have been condemned for many years, and others are recommended only to be used as a last resort. Risk assessment, widely introduced in the UK through the MHOR (1992), refined concepts of safer handling. This was reflected in *The Guide to the Handling of Patients* (Lloyd *et al.*, 1998, 4th edn), where some research evidence was quoted; however, many of the recommendations continued to be based on personal experience.

This chapter presents the evidence on controversial lifts, transfers and techniques which have been discussed in various publications over the last fifteen years as being condemned, inappropriate or presenting a risk of injury. Table 7 shows an overview of the recommendations from six publications in which the various lifts, transfers and techniques have been cited as controversial. Only three professional groups are included and we are aware that this will mean that there are omissions but hope that it will provide an overview.

The chapter is then divided into sections referring to the controversial lifts, transfers and techniques that have some research evidence for their controversial (or not) status:

- drag lift;
- shoulder lift;
- pivot lift;
- hierarchy of hazardous transfers/tasks.

3.1 DRAG LIFT

Four articles relating to the drag lift were found, two of which only commented on the incidence of the drag lift in practice. The other two studies investigated biomechanical loading. One of these is a professional opinion and the other only

Table 7 History of controversial techniques (modified from Gabbett, 1998)

Technique (alternative terminology)	Prior to 1981 (CSP, 1975)	1981 1st edn RCN (Troup et al., 1981)	1987 2nd edn RCN (Lloyd et al., 1987)	1992 3rd edn RCN (Corlett et al., 1992)	1998 (revised edn) 4th edn RCN (Lloyd et al., 1998)	1999 ASSTSAS (1999)	Derbyshire Interagency Group (2001)
Lifting	Yes	Yes – but avoid manual lifting where possible	Yes – but avoid manual lifting where possible	Yes – but never manually lift unless you have to. Place one knee on bed to get closer to patient when lifting	No – patients are never lifted manually in all but exceptional situations, or when handling babies and small children	Yes	Promotes safer handling procedures and environments
Orthodox lift (cradle, traditional) Two handlers standing on either side of the bed, lifting a patient on their clasped wrists under the patient's back and thighs. They have to lift at arms' length with a stooped and twisted posture that is only stabilised by means of a horizontal reaction between the handlers and the bed.	Yes	Avoid wherever possible as induces excessive stresses in spine and trunk	No – condemned lift as involves a stoop and a twist and breaks all rules of safe handling	No – condemned lift induces major flexion/ compression strain on lumbar spine with lateral torque during the sideways lift	No – as 1992 truncal stress of potentially injurious magnitude and 40 times more likely to cause injury than Shoulder lift (p.35) also handlers are unstable, and patient injury risk (p.226)	*	No – high risk based on MHOR weight thresholds

Technique						
Drag lift (under-arm, axilla, auxiliary, through-arm[1], hook and toss) — Refers to the method of lifting or supporting a patient by their armpits on the crooks of the carers' elbows. It is performed by two handlers to lift a patient up the bed, to carry between bed and chair, to lift off the floor, to assist standing from sitting and to support during walking.	Yes	No – condemned lift as inefficient, dangerous to handlers and often painful and brutal for the patient	No – condemned lift as 1981	No – condemned lift; biomechanically unsound for handlers, potentially harmful for patient and may provoke patient retaliation	No – condemned lift; patient and handler injury risk, dysfunctional technique, and discourages patient from mobilising	No – high risk due to taking most of patient's body weight
Walking a person linking arms — Handler and patient link arms when walking, which may result in taking weight of patient if they stumble.	*	*	*	*	*	No – high risk due to taking most of patient's body weight
Leg and arm lift (leg and arm lug) — As drag lift with handlers hooking one hand under patient's axilla and other under thighs to lift patient up in chair.	*	*	*	*	No – as drag lift, and even harder for handlers to control patient's body when sling is used	No – high risk based on MHOR weight thresholds

(continued overleaf)

Table 7 History of controversial techniques (cont.)

Technique (alternative terminology)	Prior to 1981 (CSP, 1975)	1981 1st edn RCN (Troup et al., 1981)	1987 2nd edn RCN (Lloyd et al., 1987)	1992 3rd edn RCN (Corlett et al., 1992)	1998 (revised edn) 4th edn RCN (Lloyd et al., 1998)	1999 ASSTSAS (1999)	Derbyshire Interagency Group (2001)
Shoulder lift (Australian lift) Two handlers face the bed/chair head, get close to a sitting patient and lift them on one shoulder whilst clasping the wrist of the other handler (or handling sling) under the patient's thighs. The other arm is placed on the bed (or chair arm) to act as a strut and thus reduce the stress on the spine whilst lifting the patient up the bed, or backwards from a bed into a wheelchair. Can be used by one handler with the patient using a hand block. This technique may also be used to lift and carry a sitting patient between the edge of the bed and a chair.	Yes	Yes	Yes	Last resort – and always use handling sling, though not for patients under 50 kg as it reduces handlers' leverage. Technique suitable for patients up to 50 kg	No – unsafe lift (a) truncal stress of potentially injurious magnitude and risk of cumulative strain (p.35) (b) uneven loading, shoulder strain and strut arm twisted at awkward angle which is not removed with sling use. Many patients and carers not suitable for method, and strut arm removed during transfers (p.228)	*	No – high risk based on MHOR weight thresholds

Shoulder slide Modification of the shoulder lift where a slide sheet is first introduced under the patient's buttocks. This enables handlers to slide patient up the bed and thus eliminate the lift element.	*	*	*	No – unsafe: see shoulder lift; also danger of handler lifting rather than sliding and risk of patient lifting themselves on handlers' shoulders	No – high risk based on MHOR weight thresholds
Through-arm lift[1] To lift a patient up the bed. Two handlers face bottom of bed with inside knee placed on lowered bed behind sitting patient. They place their inside arm between the patient's chest and upper arm to grasp patient's forearm, and whilst holding handling sling, placed under patient's thighs sit back on their heels to lift patient up the bed, or backwards from a bed into a wheelchair.	*	Yes	Last resort – and always use handling sling. Not recommended by one handler unless patient exceptionally light and able to assist	No – risk of injury to handlers' shoulders. Backwards transfer from bed to wheelchair incurs lifting at a distance, twisting nearly 180°, and potential for missed footing	*

(continued overleaf)

Table 7 History of controversial techniques (cont.)

Technique (alternative terminology)	Prior to 1981 (CSP, 1975)	1981 1st edn RCN (Troup et al., 1981)	1987 2nd edn RCN (Lloyd et al., 1987)	1992 3rd edn RCN (Corlett et al., 1992)	1998 (revised edn) 4th edn RCN (Lloyd et al., 1998)	1999 ASSTSAS (1999)	Derbyshire Interagency Group (2001)
Through-arm lift[1] (hammock, top and tail) To lift a patient up the bed, between bed and chair and off the floor. Taller handler is positioned behind patient in standing or half-kneeling position, and takes a through-arm grip on patient's arms (see above). Smaller handler stands at side of patient's legs to assist sideways lift into chair.	Yes	Yes	Yes – if not performed to or from a chair with high or obstructive back	Yes – last resort, and always use handling sling	No – unsafe as stooping, twisting, lifting at a distance, and uneven patient weight distribution between handlers. Risk of patient injury	Yes	No – high risk based on MHOR weight thresholds
May be performed by one handler for up bed and chair, or off-floor with patient assistance.	Yes	Yes – but only in an emergency	Yes – as 1981; three handlers with two-sling lift from floor	No – use hoist	No – use hoist. Patient assistance may unbalance lone handler during lift	*	*

Cross-arm lift

Patient is moved from bed to chair in a sitting position with a handling sling under the thighs. Two handlers face patient with their outside hand holding the sling and inside hands supporting (not lifting) under the axilla to lift and transfer to chair.

*	*	Yes	*
Yes – if patient not too heavy	*	No – unsafe Requires lifting with poor and twisted posture	*

Drawsheet lift

Drawsheet should be placed under patient from thorax to mid-thigh. Two or four handlers grasp corners of the drawsheet to help patient into sitting position and then lift up the bed. Handlers stand at side of bed or place one knee on lowered bed

Yes	*	Yes – in standing	*
Yes – one knee on lowered bed recommended	Yes – as a temporary measure	*	*

Two-sling lift (pelvic lift)

To lift the patient up the bed in a lying position using handling slings placed under the patient's hip joints and upper waist. The lift may be performed by handlers in standing position or with one knee on the bed. Alternatively can be used in crook lying to lift the pelvis for a bedpan, etc.

*	*	Yes	*
Last resort	*	No – lifting at a distance in a twisted stance. The handler's knee on the bed or the use of the sling do not adequately remove the danger	*

(continued overleaf)

Table 7 History of controversial techniques (cont.)

Technique (alternative terminology)	Prior to 1981 (CSP, 1975)	1981 1st edn RCN (Troup et al., 1981)	1987 2nd edn RCN (Lloyd et al., 1987)	1992 3rd edn RCN (Corlett et al., 1992)	1998 (revised edn) 4th edn RCN (Lloyd et al., 1998)	1999 ASSTSAS (1999)	Derbyshire Interagency Group (2001)
Combined lift This is a combination lift on a low bed. One handler uses a shoulder lift and the other faces the opposite way and places his or her inner hand under the patient's sacrum. Both handlers hold a handling sling placed under the patient's thighs.	*	*	Yes	Last resort	No – remarks as per shoulder lift apply	*	*
Three-or-more person lift Three carers stand beside bed or trolley and place their forearms underneath patient. The patient is first slid to the side, then rolled towards the carers before being lifted vertically. The trolley is then either replaced under the patient, or the shortest route taken to an adjacent one.	Yes	Yes	Yes – when no hoists, stretchers or sliding aids are available	*	No – needs perfect conditions, patient compliance and poses risk of stumbling	*	*

Technique						
Flip turn on bed Moving a patient across the bed; one or two handlers place both hands under the patient and move him or her towards them on the bed and then roll away in one movement.	Yes	*	*	*	No – unsafe; ergonomically unsound as load taken at distance from handler's body	*
Two poles and canvas lift Used to transfer patients between bed and trolley when able to stand directly behind the patient's head and without need to reach in order to grasp poles.	*	*	Yes – if helper can stand behind patient's head to avoid reaching, stooping and twisting	Yes – with spreader bars for porters and ambulance men (p56). No – lifting with arms only at waist height (p84)	*	No – high risk based on HSE weight thresholds
Front-assisted transfer with one carer (pivot transfer, elbow-lift, rocking-lift/transfer, belt holds from the front, clinging ivy, face-to-face, bear hug)	Yes	Yes	Yes	No – handlers risk of injury due to unstable posture, difficulty in controlling amount of effort required, handler linked to patient and risk of patient collapsing	Yes	No – high risk due to taking most of patient's body weight

(continued overleaf)

Table 7 History of controversial techniques (cont.)

Technique (alternative terminology)	Prior to 1981 (CSP, 1975)	1981 1st edn RCN (Troup et al., 1981)	1987 2nd edn RCN (Lloyd et al., 1987)	1992 3rd edn RCN (Corlett et al., 1992)	1998 (revised edn) 4th edn RCN (Lloyd et al., 1998)	1999 ASSTSAS (1999)	Derbyshire Interagency Group (2001)
Patient is transferred between bed and chair involving a 90° to 180° turn in a standing or half-standing position by a handler positioned in front of the patient. The main principle is to counterbalance the patient's bodyweight with the handler's bodyweight. Technique variations include foot/knee blocks, rocking, elbow/pelvic/trunk and belt hand holds. Rocking may be used to build up momentum prior to transfer, and a second carer may assist by helping the patient's buttocks round.							
Lifting with patient's arms round carer's neck during a front-assisted transfer.	*	*	*	No – condemned due to foreseeable risk of handler neck injury with passive or collapsing patient	No	*	*

Yes = recommended practice
No = identified as unsafe practice or advised against
* = no comments
1 = describes more than one technique

offers a low QR of 36 per cent. These both suggest that the use of drag lift results in forces exceeding the maximum permissible limit (MPL).

Khalil et al. (1987)

This study investigated the biomechanical load on carers' lower backs when lifting a patient:

1 two carers lifting patient from supine;
2 two carers lifting a seated patient from the edge of a chair (with patient's arms around carers' necks);
3 two carers lifting a seated patient from a chair.

The biomechanical loads were calculated from photographs using a static model. The greatest load was for Task 1, although the MPL was exceeded for both Tasks 1 and 3.

Owen et al. (1999)

This paper described a survey with nurse educators to investigate how often the axilla lift and assistive devices were (a) taught (even though not advocated in nursing text books); and (b) used in practice. Data were collected using a questionnaire (with photographs and frequency scale).

The authors found that 83 per cent of nurse educators taught the axilla lift for transferring a patient in/out of bed/chair and 56 per cent taught it for moving a patient up the bed. An even greater number observed the axilla lift being used in a clinical setting. Use of assistive devices (hydraulic lifts and gait belts) was taught and seen in use.

Owen (1999)

This paper summarised the author's previous work including the findings of a survey of nursing homes in the USA which found that 98 per cent of transfers used the drag lift. The average compressive force for this at L5/S1 exceeded the maximum recommended safety level. The author emphasised the growing body of research which points to the benefits of an ergonomic approach including assessing both patient and environmental factors.

Rodgers (1985a)

This qualitative observational study looked at the way nurses lifted and why they used those techniques.

The author found that the drag lift was the most commonly used lift with both one carer and two carers by all grades of staff. Thirty per cent of lifts were carried out by one carer even when it would have been appropriate for two. The shoulder lift was not used at all. Training in the shoulder lift did not transfer to practice on the wards.

Summary of evidence

Author and location	Subjects	Study type	QR	PR
Khalil *et al.* (1987) USA	2 nurses	x-sect.	36%	3.0
Owen *et al.* (1999) USA	368 nurse educators	survey	66%	4.0
Owen (1999) USA	—	PO	PO	4.0
Rodgers (1985a) UK	2 general medical and surgical wards (n = ?)	qual.	38%	3.5

☺☺   Limited evidence from one study that the axilla lift is still taught and used in the USA

☺☺   Limited evidence from two studies that the drag lift exceeds the maximum permissible limit (NIOSH)

3.2   SHOULDER (AUSTRALIAN) LIFT

Seven articles refer to the shoulder lift. Three of these compare it with various other lifting methods, all of which found the shoulder lift to be the least stressful, however the comparative lifts appear on the 'not recommended list' in their own right.

The study with the highest QR and PR scores investigated the shoulder lift/ slide and found that both presented a high risk of injury.

Gabbett (1998)

This M.Sc. dissertation looked at:

1   shoulder lift versus shoulder slide; and
2   shoulder slide versus a reverse slide (for moving a seated patient up the bed).

The task was evaluated using biomechanical analysis (ground reaction forces), REBA, RPE, BPDS and patient comfort. Gabbett found that there was no significant difference for using either the shoulder lift and shoulder slide, or between using the shoulder slide or the reverse slide. All were high-risk activities with respect to low-back injury.

Haigh (1993)

This study tested whether using the Australian lift, in particular the placing of feet on the bed, presented a cross-infection hazard.

No evidence was presented with respect to any connection between the Australian lift and cross-infection. So it is doubtful that nurses transferred anything to patients' beds that was highly pathogenic or not there already.

Scholey (1982)

This study looked at different ways of using a shoulder lift to see if it was effective in reducing back stress by:

1   bracing on the bed mattress;
2   holding the bed head;
3   supporting the patient's back with one hand;
4   leaving outside hand free to perform other task;
5   kneeling on the bed; and
6   using a high or low bed.

Data were collected using IAP to evaluate the above conditions.

Scholey found that there was significantly more stress when the patient's back was supported (3). The hierarchy of stress for the different methods, from the lowest to highest, was: 2:1:4:3. There was less stress if the bed was lowered so that a knee could be placed on the bed.

Stubbs and Osborne (1979)

This study evaluated the loads of activities used on a nursing shift. The authors looked at the:

1   orthodox lift;
2   three-person lift; and
3   shoulder lift.

Data were collected using an observation study, weighing of loads (direct or by comparative assessment) and IAP. They found that the orthodox lift resulted in the highest stress followed by the three-person lift with the shoulder lift generating the lowest stress. They recommended the shoulder lift as the stress was reduced by standing closer to the patient and the bracing action of the free arm.

Stubbs et al. (1983)

A two-stage study which looked at:

1   the commonly taught techniques to identify which were the least stressful with respect to loading on the back and the acceptability of the loads; and
2   whether these techniques could be successfully taught.

The four techniques were the shoulder (Australian) lift, orthodox (traditional) lift, through-arm lift, and under-arm drag. The techniques were evaluated using IAP and a five-point comfort rating scale.

The authors found that the Australian lift produced significantly lower pressures than the other three lifts, but there was no significant difference between the other three lifts. The individual subject comfort ratings were very varied, with the shoulder and orthodox lifts being more comfortable than the underarm and through-arm lifts.

Winkelmolen et al. (1994)

This study looked at the differences in working postures by calculating back compression, and collecting data on RPE for six techniques:

1   lifting up in bed with two carers;
2   shoulder lift;
3   orthodox lift;
4   barrow lift, by grasping hands under the patient's waist, with one other hand under thigh and one other hand under head;
5   through-arm lift; and
6   under-arm lift.

The authors recorded the working posture in terms of:

- flexion, lateral flexion and rotation;
- the biomechanical stress as the compressive force relative to the maximum permissive load; and
- the subjective stress as RPE and body-part discomfort.

The results found that the barrow lift caused significantly more stress than the shoulder or orthodox lifts, and that the orthodox and barrow lifts produced more subjective stress than the under-arm and through-arm lifts. The shoulder lift was the least stressful.

Wright (1981a and b)

These papers gave a professional opinion and described a general investigation into handling techniques in nursing. Data were collected by the observation of patients and equipment in theatres; lifting patients after total hip replacement.

The Australian lift was not seen to be used at all. Wright recommended increased use of lifts and equipment and wearing trousers as part of the uniform.

Summary of evidence

Author and location	Subjects	Study type	QR	PR
Gabbett (1998) UK	57 student nurses	expt	63%	4.5
Haigh (1993) UK	nurses (n = ?)	survey	52%	5.0
Scholey (1982) UK	2 female subjects	quasi	41%	4.0
Stubbs and Osborne (1979) UK	4 nurses	quasi	31%	4.0
Stubbs et al. (1983) UK	8 nurses	quasi	59%	4.5
Wright (1981a and b) UK	2 hospitals (n = ?)	x-sect.	11%	2.0
Winkelmolen et al. (1994) Netherlands	10 female subjects (not nurses)	quasi	63%	4.5

☺☺☺   Moderate evidence from three studies that the shoulder lift presents less of a risk than the orthodox lift, through-arm lift, under-arm drag or barrow lift

☺☺   Limited evidence from one study that the shoulder slide has the same level of risk as the shoulder lift and that both are high-risk techniques

☺☺   Limited evidence from one study that the shoulder lift does not increase cross-infection risks

3.3   PIVOT LIFT

Only one, high-quality quasi-experiment was found referring to the pivot lift. It shows that the pivot transfer presents a higher risk than any of the two-carer transfers investigated.

Marras et al. *(1999)*

This study aimed to identify the nature and range of low-back spinal forces and risk of low-back disorder associated with the various patient-handling tasks and techniques.

Table 8 Tasks and technique options (Marras *et al.*, 1999)

Tasks	Technique options
Bed–wheelchair with two arms	One-carer hug
Bed–wheelchair with one arm	Two-carer hook and toss (measured for both right and left carer)
Commode–hospital room chair	Two-carer with gait belt

Outcome measures included an EMG-assisted biomechanical model; LMM; and bipolar electrodes at the ten major trunk muscle sites.

The authors found that the single-carer hug method resulted in about 10 per cent higher risk than any of the two-carer transferring methods, with lifting from the hospital chair having the highest risk and compression values. The use of the gait belt only reduced the loading for the carer positioned on the right side of the patient. None of the transfers was considered hazardous to use in a hospital setting for either one or two carers. Both the biomechanical model and EMG results indicated that all the lifting techniques had a high probability of being in the high-risk group.

Summary of evidence

Author and location	Subjects	Study type	QR	PR
Marras *et al.* (1999) USA	12 experienced and 5 inexperienced patient handlers	quasi	72%	5.0

☺☺　　Limited evidence from one study that the pivot lift presents a higher risk than two-carer transfers

3.4　HIERARCHY OF HAZARDOUS TRANSFERS/TASKS

The remaining thirteen studies collected on controversial issues have been grouped together as they identify risks inherent in some tasks rather than referring to specific techniques.

Bell (1979)

This survey collected information on five major patient-lifting tasks for which manual handling was most often used. These tasks involved transfers to/from:

1 bed;
2 bath;
3 chair;
4 toilet; and
5 repositioning.

Data were collected using a questionnaire. Each task was considered to be of equal importance to patient care and two members of staff were generally considered to be needed for lifting.

The physical effort involved for the tasks was rated as being high. The bath and bed tasks involved the greatest number of patients but were less frequently undertaken than the other tasks. Hoists were used for bathing patients on 23 per cent of occasions although manual lifting with two members of staff was the most common technique. No detailed information was given about the specific techniques used for the tasks.

Dehlin et al. (1976)

This study investigated whether the lifting technique (knee action or derrick action) showed any relationship to the occurrence of low-back symptoms.

The authors examined three tasks:

1 turning a patient on one side in bed;
2 sliding a patient up in bed towards the pillows; and
3 giving lift assistance during transfer from bed to chair.

Data were collected using a questionnaire. Sixty-five per cent of subjects adopted a knees-bent and body-stooped posture for all three tasks, representing a mid-stance posture between the knee and derrick actions.

Garg et al. (1992)

This survey collected data on patient-handling tasks to establish a hierarchy of perceived stress. Sixteen task categories were ranked for stressfulness using RPE. These were then observed to carry out postural analysis using a biomechanical model.

The authors found that the toileting process was ranked as the most stressful task, whereas making an empty bed was the least stressful. Manual lifting (hook and toss, drag lift) was used 98 per cent of the time for patients needing help. The manual hoist took approximately 180 seconds to use in comparison with the manual method, which took 18 seconds. They reported that even lifting

25th-percentile-weight patients exceeded the limit recommended by NIOSH (1981). The conclusion was that the strength requirements of the nursing assistant's job were so great that education and training on body mechanics and lifting technique alone would not reduce the high prevalence of low-back pain.

Green (1996)

This qualitative study observed moving and handling practices on two medical wards to explore nurses' perceptions of factors that might influence moving and handling practices. Thirty hours of observational data were collected over a five-day period. Factors included: space in the design and layout of the workplace, in particular the bed-side and toilet areas; management of nursing care (time and equipment use); training sessions; consistency of moving and handling practice; use of unsafe techniques; attitude of colleagues; availability of equipment; documentation; and design of uniforms.

Green concluded that attitudes had a strong influence on moving and handling practice, in particular the influence of other team members: nurses did not want to risk becoming unpopular and so would carry out unsafe moving and handling practice alone.

Harber et al. (1987)

This paper carried out a survey to characterise the work actually performed by nurses in order to determine those actions which were frequent and likely to contribute to back pain. They used an activity-observation system to record:

- duration of the posture;
- body position (upright, squat, semi-squat);
- starting and stopping location; and
- nature of the activity (push, pull, etc.) and other information.

The findings indicated that most patient-movement actions were performed in bed (sit up, roll side-to-side), accounting for 10.7 out of 16.5 transfers per shift. However, non-patient activities were more frequent than patient activities.

Hui et al. (2001)

The authors compared subjective rating (RPE) and objective measures (heart rate and thirty-minute log of patient-care activities) of nursing activities in a geriatric setting.

Hui et al. found that turning patients, solo transfers and showering recorded heart rates of 127–129 bpm, and RPE of 15–17 in comparison with shared transfer and changing pads/sheets at 95–118 bpm and 11–12 RPE. They suggested that this gave a hierarchy of task difficulty although only two female nurses were used.

Kato et al. (2000)

This study analysed a bear hug/pivot (with one carer) for a paralysed patient to transfer from wheelchair to sitting on a bed with respect to the position of the wheelchair. The wheelchair was positioned at:

1   the head of the bed; and
2   the foot of the bed.

The authors found that the transfer was quicker with the wheelchair at the foot of the bed.

Laflin and Aja (1995)

This study looked at three different techniques to carry out a bed-to-chair transfer:

1   side-to-side;
2   top–tail; and
3   crossed arm.

The authors evaluated the lifts using:

• the NIOSH lifting formula to compare with the lifting index;
• the Bloswick measure of compressive force; and
• the Genaidy formula (see original paper for more details).

The results showed that the positions for the staff for all techniques exceeded the maximum guidelines for all three outcome measures.

Love (1996a)

This study investigated:

1   the specific accounts of work-injured nurses to see whether a common factor existed which could become the target of preventive measures; and
2   whether lifting in bed or out of bed was more hazardous.

Data were collected using a questionnaire to ask about both the injury and the circumstances of the lifting injury.

Love found that 86 per cent had been injured as a result of lifting patients, all resulting in back injuries. Most occurred at a busy time of shift, with eighteen occurring during out-of-bed activities and nine when moving patients in bed. She concluded that assisting when the patient was out of bed or getting out of bed was significantly more likely to lead to injury than when the patient was in bed.

Owen (1987)

The author reported two studies carried out to describe back problems in nursing and to elicit ideas from the nurses for preventive approaches. She sent postal questionnaires to 570 registered nurses in Wisconsin, USA to collect data about the factors precipitating the onset of back pain.

The authors found that 62 per cent of episodes of back pain were perceived to have been precipitated by moving a patient in bed.

Table 9 Data from Owen (1987)

Task	Number (and percentage) of back-pain episodes	
	Study 1	Study 2
Manoeuvring a patient in bed	319 (62%)	128 (58%)
Transferring patient between bed/cart/chair	92 (18%)	62 (25%)
Stabilising a patient from falling	27 (5%)	22 (9%)
Restraining a patient	23 (4%)	8 (3%)
Non-patient-handling tasks	52 (11%)	24 (10%)

The manoeuvring-in-bed tasks were then sub-divided into:

- lifting, pulling and sliding up in bed (53 per cent);
- turning a patient (29 per cent);
- repositioning a patient (9 per cent);
- positioning a patient up to the side of the bed (5 per cent);
- lifting a patient's head (2 per cent);
- bed bathing (2 per cent); and
- CPR (0.5 per cent).

In both studies nursing personnel tended to look at back problems in reference to changes they should make themselves (e.g. good body mechanics, asking for help), rather than looking at external factors of organisation or design.

Owen et al. (1992)

This study described four methods to identify (comparison and ranking) the most back-stressing tasks performed by nursing assistants in a nursing home. They identified 153 tasks which were grouped into sixteen task categories. The outcome measures included: RPE; comparative ranking for stressfulness; postural measurement for the compression force on L5/S1; 3D static biomechanical model to estimate the tensile strength on the erector spinae muscles.

The authors found that the most stressful tasks involved transferring patients from one destination to another: toileting (toilet to and from chair); bed transfers (bed to and from chair); and bathing. The most practical method to identify back-stressing tasks was RPE. It was the easiest to administer and essentially identified the same tasks as those identified by the other methods.

Schibye and Skotte (2000)

This study looked at the working postures and mechanical load on the low back during the most common patient-handling tasks and then compared the variation in the load between the different tasks with the variation in load between the subjects when they performed the same task. All the tasks were manual, performed by a single carer with a left hemiplegic (stroke) patient on a height-adjustable bed:

1   turning in bed from supine to left-side lying (towards carer);
2   repositioning from the middle of the bed to the nearest bedside;
3   turning from supine to right-side lying (away from carer);
4   elevating from supine in bed to sitting on the edge of the bed;
5   lifting the patient from sitting on the edge of the bed to standing;
6   moving from sitting to a supine position in bed;
7   transferring from sitting on the bed to sitting in a wheelchair;
8   positioning backwards in the seat of the wheelchair; and
9   repositioning higher upwards in bed.

The working postures and mechanical load were measured using a 3D bio-mechanical dynamic multi-segment model for L4/5 with two force plates to stand on at the edge of the bed; EMG of erector spinae; LMM to measure the kinematics of the low back.

The authors found that there was high inter-subject variation for all the outcome variables for a given task, so the exposure assessment should include an individual measure for risk. The highest-risk moments were identified as being during the two tasks typically involving a lifting procedure of the whole body weight: (5: lifting from sitting on the edge of the bed to standing and 8: repositioning backwards in a wheelchair); but also for two repositioning tasks: (2: repositioning from the middle of the bed to the nearest side to the carer; and 9: repositioning higher upwards in the bed).

Smedley et al. (1995)

This study reported a survey to examine the risk of back symptoms in nurses in relation to a range of lifting tasks. It used a postal questionnaire to give a self-reported estimate of the number of times each subject performed each of a series of patient-handling tasks per average shift. The associations between low-back pain and risk factors were assessed by logistics regression to give risk estimates at 95 per cent confidence intervals.

The findings suggested that the pattern of risk was consistent with bio-mechanical evaluation. Three tasks presented an increased risk with respect to low-back pain:

1   manually moving a patient around on a bed;
2   transferring from a bed to chair; and
3   lifting a patient from the floor.

Summary of evidence

Author and location	Subjects	Study type	QR	PR
Bell (1979) UK	725 wards in 85 hospitals	survey	82%	3.5
Dehlin et al. (1976) Sweden	267 nursing aides	survey	75%	4.0
Garg et al. (1992) USA	38 nursing assistants	survey	55%	4.5
Green (1996) UK	5 nurses, 3 health-care assistants, 2 nursing students	qual.	31%	3.0
Harber et al. (1987) USA	63 nurses	survey	55%	4.0
Hui et al. (2001) Hong Kong	2 nurses	x-sect.	66%	4.0
Kato et al. (2000) Japan	2 nurses	survey	32%	2.0
Laflin and Aja (1995) USA	2 nurses	quasi	46%	4.0
Love (1996a) UK	41 nurses	survey	36%	4.0
Owen (1987) USA	570 nurses	survey	45%	4.0
Owen et al. (1992) USA	38 nursing assistants	x-sect.	82%	4.0
Schibye and Skotte (2000) Denmark	10 female nurses	quasi	65%	4.0
Smedley et al. (1995) UK	2405 nurses	survey	82%	4.0

☺☺☺   Moderate evidence from seven studies that the most hazardous tasks involve: moving patients in bed; bed–chair transfers; toileting; bathing; and lifting from the floor

☺☹   Limited evidence from one study that nurses worked in stooped postures

SECTION II

PATIENT-HANDLING TASKS

CHAPTER 4

TRANSFERS

4.1   TRANSFERS STARTING FROM A LYING POSITION

This chapter is divided into sections looking at different types of transfers to give a practical grouping of the papers. The introduction to each section lists methods that have been suggested in professional guidelines for carrying out the transfer. The information has been compiled from the following sources: Disabled Living Foundation (2001); Essex Group of National Back Exchange (1996); The Disability Information Trust (1996); Royal College of Midwives (1997); Lloyd *et al.* (National Back Pain Association/Royal College of Nursing, 1998, revised edition); South London and Kent Group, National Back Exchange (1998); Health Services Advisory Committee (1998); Chartered Society of Physiotherapy (1998); Oxford Region, National Back Exchange (1999); ASSTSAS (1999); Human Services/Victorian Work cover Authority (1999); Graham *et al.* (2000); The Resuscitation Council (2001); Derbyshire Interagency Group (2001). The detail of each technique is not given here so we recommend that you refer to the original publications for further information.

The flow charts in Chapters 4 and 5 have three action boxes:

1   Hands Off: by supervision and verbal prompts and/or providing equipment to facilitate completely independent movement by the patient;
2   Hands On (some help): giving assistance using manual techniques and/or equipment with the patient assisting the movement, transfer, care or repositioning task;
3   Hands On (a lot of help): moving dependent patients who are assessed as mostly unable or unsuitable to give assistance (e.g. non-weight-bearing and/or uncooperative).

4.1.1 Lying to lying

Transferring from a lying position to a lying position can include a variety of starting places, including the floor, beds, trolleys, stretchers, treatment plinths, examination couches, x-ray tables, operating tables, mortuary tables/fridges, etc. Four studies were found which looked at this task. Only one study had a QR score of ≥50 per cent, so an evidence statement in the limited category is given. The other studies had QR scores of less than 50 per cent, but did not investigate the same questions, so their evidence cannot be combined to support a statement.

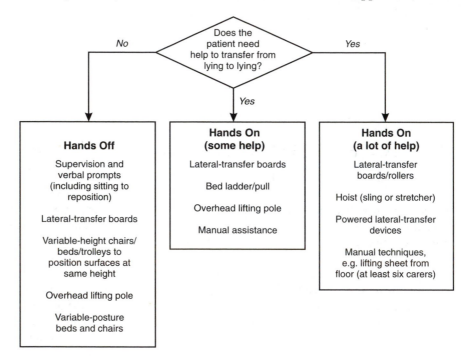

Figure 2 Transfers from lying to lying

Suggestions from professional guidelines (not exhaustive)

Dolan and Adams (1998)

A study evaluating the effectiveness of various assistive aids and hoists in reducing the peak bending and compressive stresses acting on the lumbar spine. There were five tasks and three conditions. This section includes the bed–trolley transfer which was carried out using:

1   a lateral transfer board and full-length transfer sheet; and
2   a hoist.

Spinal compression was measured with EMG of the back muscles, spinal bending was measured as spinal curvature using an electromagnetic motion analysis device over L5/S1.

The results showed that the time taken was substantially increased when using the aids; however, there was no significant difference in the time-dependent compression and flexion so aids may take longer but are not necessarily more harmful. The effectiveness of the hoist only reduced peak compression loading by 5–23 per cent as it required nurses to adopt awkward, stooped postures while securing and positioning the patient in the hoist.

Ng et al. (1997)

In this survey fifty-five junior doctors were asked about their approach to lifting a patient with a dense stroke up off the floor. The telephone survey asked about:

- the methods of lifting used;
- the outcome of the lift;
- any musculoskeletal-related injury and training/instruction received.

All said that they would try to lift a dense stroke patient but none described a safe approach. Seventy-three per cent (38) had tried to lift patients alone, and 19 per cent (10) had sustained a back injury as a result (eight were female). Only 50 per cent (26) had received lifting instruction, but 94 per cent (49) thought that specific training would be helpful.

Revie (2000)

This study looked at moving and handling of the deceased in the funeral industry. It described a risk assessment which recommended: redesign of premises; re-design of working practices; use of trolleys and hoists; removal of carpets or putting larger wheels on trolleys; using a single-tray system in mortuary; height-adjustable trolleys for fridge–table transfers.

Zelenka et al. (1996)

An analysis of the efficiency, with respect to the force required, of commercially available transfer devices suitable for the task of a lateral horizontal transfer between a bed and trolley (gurney) was undertaken. The three devices were:

1 a patient roller: a frame of five rollers with a plasticised cover which is rolled under the patient as they are pulled between the surfaces;
2 a patient shifter: a thin, semi-rigid plastic board with four handles cut along each side. The patient is moved with patient shifter between surfaces, so is not a bridging board;
3 a drawsheet.

Four hundred and fifty transfers were carried out with the three devices. Force scales were used to obtain the maximum forces required.

Results showed that the patient roller required consistently lower force (44 per cent less) than the shifter or drawsheet regardless of the direction of force applied. The patient shifter, in turn, required less force than the drawsheet. The patient roller was recommended.

Summary of evidence

Author and location	Subjects	Study type	QR	PR
Dolan et al. (1998) UK	25 female nurses	quasi	48%	5.0
Ng et al. (1997) UK	55 junior hospital doctors	survey	52%	5.0
Revie (2000) UK	–	PO	PO	2.5
Zelenka et al. (1996) USA	15 hospital workers and office staff	quasi	48%	3.5

☺☹   Limited evidence from one study showed that doctors would like moving and handling training on moving patients from the floor

4.1.2   Lying to sitting

Four studies were found which looked at this task. Most of the equipment and techniques in Figure 3 do not appear in the research literature. This limits the conclusion and recommendations which can be drawn for practice. All four studies had QR scores of less than 50 per cent. They investigated different research questions so the evidence cannot be combined into a statement.

Bertolazzi and Saia (1999)

An assessment of the risk to staff of transferring uncooperative or partially cooperative patients with respect to the environmental assessment and provision of aids:

1   from bed to stretcher;
2   moving in bed.

The assessment was made using a checklist on forty-nine medical wards, fifty-three surgical wards and twenty-three health-care areas and twenty-one service/diagnostic/emergency areas in eight hospitals. The checklist included an analysis

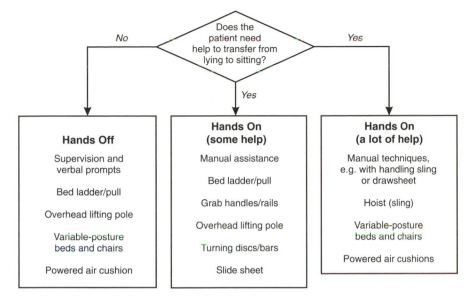

Figure 3 Transfers from lying to sitting
Suggestions from professional guidelines (not exhaustive)

of the work organisation and environment, and the availability of aids, space, types of beds and number of non-self-sufficient patients.

The authors found that medical wards had the highest risk value (61 per cent) especially if they had elderly patients. The greatest risks were transferring from bed to stretcher and moving the patient in the bed. There was inadequate space in 50 per cent of the wards. The easiest bed to move was an adjustable-height bed with four directional wheels.

DeGeorge and Dunwoody (1995)

This informal survey was carried out with six orthopaedic surgeons to explore the preferred way of lifting the lower extremity with an external fixator for a bed–chair transfer.

The recommendation depended on the condition of the patient, but the safest way was to support the fixator itself, though some surgeons were concerned that repeated manipulations of the frame might loosen the pin and fracture alignment.

Dolan and Adams (1998)

This study evaluated the effectiveness of various assistive aids and hoists in reducing the peak bending and compressive stresses acting on the lumbar spine. There were five tasks and three conditions. This section looks at the task of lying to sitting using three techniques:

1   shoulder lift;

2   shoulder slide with short transfer sheet with handles;
3   reverse through-arm slide using short transfer sheet with handles;
4   hoist.

Spinal compression was measured with EMG of the back muscles (with allowance for muscle length and contraction velocity). Spinal bending was measured as spinal curvature using an electromagnetic motion analysis device over L5/S1.

It was found that the sliding tasks tended to mimic manual tasks. The time taken was substantially increased when using the aids; however, there was no significant difference in the time-dependent compression and flexion, so aids may take longer but are not necessarily more harmful. The effectiveness of the hoist only reduced peak compression loading by 5–23 per cent as it required nurses to adopt awkward, stooped postures while securing and positioning the patient in the hoist.

Khalil et al. (1987)

This study aimed to calculate the biomechanical stresses incurred on a nurse's lower back while lifting a patient:

1   sitting up in bed from lying;
2   standing from sitting on the edge of the bed;
3   standing up from a chair.

The study calculated the force on the erector spinae, reactive force on L5/S1 and found that standing from a chair gave most load to nurses; however, sitting from lying supine gave the most reactive force at L5/S1.

Summary of evidence

Author and location	Subjects	Study type	QR	PR
Bertolazzi and Saia (1999) Italy	health-care workers at 8 hospitals (n = ?)	survey	25%	2.0
DeGeorge and Dunwoody (1995) USA	6 orthopaedic surgeons	survey	18%	2.5
Dolan et al. (1998) UK	25 female nurses	quasi	48%	5.0
Khalil et al. (1987) USA	2 nurses	quasi	7%	3.5

☹   Poor or no evidence to support any of the techniques or equipment as
recommended in the professional guidelines

4.2   TRANSFERS FROM A SEATED POSITION

This section presents the literature which explored the task of transferring a
patient from a sitting position to another sitting position. This could include any
combination of the following starting and finishing positions: bed, chair, wheelchair, toilet, shower chair, commode, car seat, floor, trolley, etc.

4.2.1   Sitting to sitting

Seventeen studies were found looking at this transfer. There was moderate
evidence provided by consistent findings from three studies that mechanical aids
should be used for dependent (non-weight-bearing patients). There was also
moderate evidence for using a walking belt with two carers from five studies. The
use of two carers with a walking belt was reinforced by three studies which found
that using a walking belt with one carer (from the front) was unsafe. For the other
equipment mentioned in the professional guidance (Figure 4 on page 52) no
research was found from this search. Other studies are listed as giving limited
evidence if they had a QR score of ≥50 per cent but were unsupported by other
work (single study). These include sliding techniques, using a gantry hoist and a
comparative evaluation of patient rollers.

Benevolo et al. (1993)

This study looked at five methods of transferring a patient between a bed and a
wheelchair:

1   manual method with one carer (stand in front, lock knees, grip patient by
    arms/armpits, lift and transfer);
2   manual method with two carers (stand at the side of the patient, grip under
    armpits and elbows, lift and transfer);
3   walking belt with one carer (hold handles on walking belt, block knees,
    rock, pull and transfer);
4   walking belt with two carers (stand to front/side, block foot, bend knees,
    grip belt and stabilise with other hand on wheelchair, rock, pull, lift and
    transfer);
5   mechanical hoist (chains and slings).

The outcome measures included RPE; perceived safety (by patient and nurse);
patient comfort; preferential ranking of transfer type by carer; time for each
transfer.

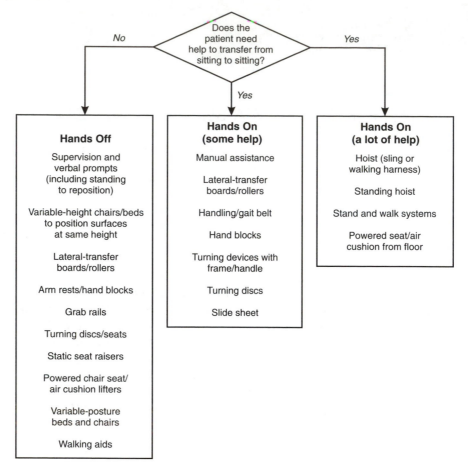

Figure 4 Transfers from sitting to sitting

Suggestions from professional guidelines (not exhaustive)

The authors found that the walking belt with two carers was the most efficient for all the measures, followed by the mechanical hoist and walking belt with one carer.

Dehlin and Lindberg (1975)

This study aimed to determine the lifting burden of a nursing aide, measured as the vertical force in the foot plane (using a force plate) and time taken when giving lift assistance to a number of patients. Three different lifts were investigated:

1   sliding a patient up in bed towards the pillows;
2   giving assistance to the patient during the transfer from bed to chair;
3   giving assistance to the patient during the transfer from chair to bed.

The bed height was varied and Tasks 2 and 3 were performed using a bear-hug lift or a bear hug (pivot).

The authors found that most lifts took less than twenty seconds and the nurses could not get into ideal postures (knees bent/back straight). There was a significant correlation between the patient body-weight and the vertical force on the force plate, with the maximum recommendation from the ILO (22 kg) being exceeded several times during the study.

Dolan and Adams (1998)

This study evaluated the effectiveness of various assistive aids and hoists in reducing the peak bending and compressive stresses acting on the lumbar spine. There were five tasks and three conditions. This section includes the data on bed-to-chair and toileting tasks using the following techniques.

Bed-to-chair:

1   through-arm lift with reverse hold;
2   reverse through-arm slide with short transfer sheet and lateral-transfer board; and
3   hoist.

Toileting:

1   manual handling belt; and
2   standing hoist.

Spinal compression was measured with EMG of the back muscles (with allowance for muscle length and contraction velocity). Spinal bending was measured as spinal curvature using an an electromagnetic motion analysis device over L5/S1.

The results showed that sliding tasks tended to mimic manual tasks. The time taken was substantially increased when using the aids; however, there was no significant difference in the time-dependent compression and flexion so aids may take longer but are not necessarily more harmful. Various aids significantly reduced the peak- and time-dependent loading of the lumbar spine but only by a modest amount. The effectiveness of the hoist only reduced peak-compression loading by 5–23 per cent as it required nurses to adopt awkward, stooped postures while securing and positioning the patient in the hoist.

Elford et al. (2000)

This quasi-experiment investigated whether the use of patient-handling slings for lifting a patient from one seat to another reduced the risk of injury to the lumbar spine, compared to a similar technique without slings. Both one-sling and two-sling techniques were examined. Outcome measures were angular displacement and velocity, measured with a lumbar motion monitor, and body-part stress-rating. Angular displacement showed lower values for both one and two slings than for no slings. Since the sling effectively lengthens the carer's arm, the amount of trunk flexion decreased. However the experiment only measured angles and not forces, so could not be applied to reducing the risk of injury. Subjectively the subjects preferred one or two slings to none.

Gagnon et al. (1986)

This study looked at three methods of raising a patient from a chair with one carer:

1   with the hands;
2   with forearms behind the patient's back at shoulder level;
3   with a belt held at waist level.

The forces acting on the lumbar spine at L5/S1 were estimated using EMG (erector spinae and oblique externals), video, force platform and measurement of the lever arm from photographs. The authors found that the technique with the belt (3) was the most strenuous with respect to compressive forces, whereas the manual technique (1) had the lowest compression forces. The use of the belt was associated with higher levels of both internal and external work than the other two methods due to the different motion pattern characteristics at the beginning of the move and the longer lifting time.

Gagnon and Lortie (1987)

This paper describes three studies. This section includes the information about lifting from a chair with one carer:

1   forearms behind patient's back; and
2   belt grasped at waist level.

They used biomechanical modelling with force plates for the feet and knees; EMG; and cinematography to record motions and calculated net reactions at L5/S1.
    The results showed that the method using the belt should not be used with one carer as it resulted in a higher peak compression force.

Garg et al. (1991a)

This laboratory study looked at the task of transferring a patient from a shower chair to a wheelchair using eight different techniques. Five manual methods were used:

1   lifting with two carers (drag);
2   rocking and pulling the patient with a gait belt (5 cm wide, no handles) and
    two carers;

3   rocking and pulling the patient with a sling (flexible polymer, 20.5 cm long, 50 cm wide with cut-outs for handles at each end) and one carer;
4   rocking and pulling the patient with a walking belt (12.5 cm, handles on each side) and one carer;
5   rocking and pulling the patient with a walking belt and two carers.

Three different makes of mechanical hoists were used. The outcome measures included: biomechanical evaluations, RPE, comfort and security ratings for patients; suitability of method for patients condition; carer's overall preference; transfer time.

The authors found that patients preferred the pulling techniques (except the gait belt) as they were more comfortable than lifting. The walking belt with two carers was the preferred method. Two of the hoists were perceived to be more stressful than the walking belt with one or two carers. Their recommendation was to use:

- the walking belt with two carers and a gentle rocking/pulling motion for weight-bearing patients;
- one of the hoists for non-weight-bearing, heavy or combative patients;
- a wheelchair for a to/from shower chair transfer.

Garg et al. (1991b)

This laboratory study looked at the task of transferring a patient from a bed to a wheelchair using eight different techniques. Five manual methods were used:

1   lifting with two carers (drag);
2   rocking and pulling the patient with a gait belt (5 cm wide, no handles) and two carers;
3   rocking and pulling the patient with a sling (flexible polymer, 20.5 cm long, 50 cm wide with cut-outs for handles at each end) and one carer;
4   rocking and pulling the patient with a walking belt (12.5 cm, handles on each side) and one carer;
5   rocking and pulling the patient with a walking belt and two carers.

Three different makes of mechanical hoists were used. The outcome measures included: biomechanical evaluations (body angles, pulling forces), nine-point RPE scale, comfort and security ratings for patients; suitability of method for patients condition; carer's overall preference; transfer time.

The authors found that the use of a mechanical aid did not necessarily reduce stress as two of the hoists took longer than some of the manual techniques. Their recommendation was to use:

- the walking belt with two carers and a gentle rocking/pulling motion for weight-bearing patients;
- one of the hoists for non-weight-bearing, heavy or combative patients.

Garg and Owen (1994)

This study looked at transfers between toilet and wheelchair using eight different methods (five manual methods):

1   lifting with two carers (drag);
2   rocking and pulling the patient with a gait belt (5 cm wide, no handles) and two carers;
3   rocking and pulling the patient with a sling (flexible polymer, 20.5 cm long, 50 cm wide with cut-outs for handles at each end) and one carer;
4   rocking and pulling the patient with a walking belt (12.5 cm, handles on each side) and one carer;
5   rocking and pulling the patient with a walking belt and two carers;
6–8   three different makes of mechanical hoists were used.

The authors evaluated the biomechanical stress using five measures in the laboratory: Body Part Discomfort Chart; RPE; biomechanical modelling from a video; time for transfer to be achieved; and subjective opinions on safety, comfort and personal preference from both carer and patient perspectives. The field study looked at RPE, injury statistics and acceptability, based on actual usage. The patients were classified into three groups based on their physical ability.

The authors' recommendation was the walking belt with two carers. Two of the hoists were perceived to be more stressful, less comfortable and less secure to use than the walking belt with two carers.

Gingher et al. (1996)

This randomised, controlled trial looked at the Assist Personal Transfer System (a gantry hoist) compared with a mobile hoist (lift) and manual lifting. Two long-term care facilities were used giving thirty-three residents and fifty-two nursing aides as subjects. The outcome measures included the number of lifts, number of staff needed, number of lifts per shift, and the amount of time per lift.

The results showed that manual lifting was faster than hoisting, with no difference between mobile and gantry hoists. Residents appeared to respond better to the gantry hoist. The gantry hoist was used more than the mobile hoist. The recommendation was that overhead/gantry hoists were better than mobile hoists for bed-to-chair transfers.

Kothiyal and Yven (2000)

This quasi-experiment evaluated the muscle strain experienced by nursing staff during the transfer of a patient from a shower chair to a low chair with and without using a handling sling. Muscular strain was measured using EMG to erector spinae, although exactly how and where the electrodes were applied was not clear. Also an RPE scale was used to gauge subject perception.

The authors found that the use of a handling sling did not lead to any significant difference in muscle activity of erector spinae or trapezius (left or right) and there was a significant increase in perceived exertion on shoulder and lower back when the device was used. They recommended that patient-handling aids should be adjustable and attention should be given to the anthropometry of users.

Marras et al. (1999)

This study aimed to identify the nature and range of low-back spinal forces and risk of low-back disorder associated with the various patient-handling tasks and techniques. Outcome measures included an EMG-assisted biomechanical model and LMM.

Table 10 Task details from Marras et al. (1999)

Tasks	Technique options
Bed–wheelchair with two arms	One-carer hug
Bed–wheelchair with one arm	Two-carer hook and toss (measured for both right and left carer)
Commode–hospital room chair	Two-carer with gait belt

The authors found that the single-carer hug method resulted in about 10 per cent higher risk than any of the two-carer transferring methods, with lifting from the hospital chair having the highest risk and compression values. The use of the gait belt reduced the loading only for the carer positioned on the right side of the patient. None of the transfers was considered hazardous to use in a hospital setting for either one or two carers. Both the biomechanical model and EMG indicated that all the lifting techniques had a high probability of being in the high-risk group.

Owen and Fragala (1999)

This study compared the perceived physical exertion experienced by nursing staff in using three different techniques to transfer from bed to chair:

1   stretcher chair (chair which converts from a chair into a stretcher) and transfer pad;
2   gait belt; and
3   hoist.

The outcome measures used RPE and patient comfort and security.
    The authors found that Option 1 resulted in significantly less stress than the traditional methods (gait belt and hoist). Removing the transfer pad was the most difficult activity. The patients also reported feeling significantly more comfortable and secure.

Roth et al. (1993)

This quasi-experiment looked at the use of a belt lifter (stand-and-raise aid, standing hoist) for changing incontinence briefs, toileting and bed–chair transfers in comparison with manual methods. The outcome measures included a questionnaire undertaken after five months to collect data on preference, perceived level of exertion, likelihood of use and level of helpfulness.

The results showed that nursing staff preferred the belt lifter for all manoeuvres and that the time taken did not increase significantly compared to manual methods.

Ulin et al. (1997)

This study looked at transfers from bed to wheelchair for two totally dependent patients (light and heavy weights) using six methods, all performed with two carers:

1   pivot transfer;
2   gait belt;
3   sliding board;
4   screw-actuated lift;
5   hydraulic lift; and
6   electric lift.

The outcome measures included RPE; compressive force on L5/S1 using a 3D static strength prediction programme; force gauge to determine the force required to roll or position patient and pump the hoist; hand force; and posture modelling.

The authors found that low-back compressive forces exceeded the back compression NIOSH limits for manual methods but not mechanical methods. No difference was found in RPE between light and heavy patients for manual methods. They predicted that less than 4 per cent of the female population would have the strength at the hip to perform the transfer using the gait belt, and for all the manual methods less than 53 per cent of the female population would have sufficient strength to carry out the transfer. They recommended that mechanical lifts should be used to transfer totally dependent patients from a bed to wheelchair regardless of patient weight.

Zhuang et al. (1999)

This study looked at a sitting transfer from a bed to chair with respect to biomechanical stress on carers using twelve different transfer methods:

1   manual method with two carers (baseline measurements);
2   walking belt with two carers;
3   sliding board with one carer;

4–7   stand-up lift with one carer (four different makes/models);
8   overhead lift with one carer;
9–12 basket-sling lifter with one carer (four different makes/models).

The outcome measures included: body postures and joint angles (3D motion analysis); ground reaction forces (force platforms); L5/S1 compressive force (3D biomechanical model); percentage of the population with sufficient strength to perform task.

Transferring patients between bed and chair was found to be very stressful for some carers even when assistive devices were used. The authors found a significant difference in manoeuvring force relating to the design of the wheels, width and length of base and location of pushing frame. A significant difference was also found in the force to pull the sling handle due to the design of sling, sling handle and handle position and frame of lift to give a difference in force required to pull patients into sitting position. In the preparation stage before the transfer the manual lift, walking belt, sliding board and stand-up lift all exceeded the maximum NIOSH recommended limit for back compressive forces. Their recommendation was to use the basket sling and overhead lift as they significantly reduced the biomechanical load on the carer's back.

Zhuang et al. (2000)

Using the same transfer methods as in their 1999 study, the authors looked at a sitting transfer from a bed to chair with respect to psychophysical stress on carers. The outcome measures included: RPE; rating scale for ease of use, ranking preference of methods; patient ranking for comfort and security; and time for task.

The authors' recommended methods were a walking belt, two of the stand-up lifts and two of the basket lifts. The walking belt was faster than the mechanical equipment. All were equivalent for comfort and security.

4.2.2   Sitting to standing

The four studies in this section give limited evidence from one high-quality study that transfers with patients weighing less than 16.9 kg may be safe. Two of the studies (one with a high QR) give limited evidence that the walking harness (hoist) and standing hoist are suitable equipment for use in early rehabilitation.

Busse (2000)

This study looked at the use of hoists in rehabilitation using a functional impendence measure to assess the patient's initial dependency. The equipment used for the rehabilitation programme was:

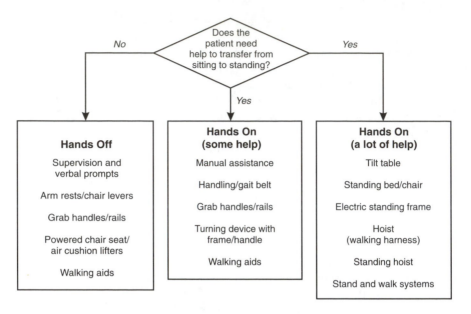

Figure 5 Transfers from sitting to standing

Suggestions from professional guidelines (not exhaustive)

Summary of evidence

Author and location	Subjects	Study type	QR	PR
Benevolo *et al.* (1993) Italy	6 nurses and 6 physiotherapists	quasi	57%	4.0
Dehlin and Lindberg (1975) Sweden	1 nursing aide	quasi	63%	3.0
Dolan *et al.* (1998) UK	25 female nurses	quasi	48%	5.0
Elford *et al.* (2000) Australia	23 nurses	quasi	76%	3.5
Gagnon and Lortie (1987) Canada	15 nursing aides	quasi	35%	4.0
Gagnon *et al.* (1986) Canada	6 male nursing students	quasi	57%	4.0
Garg *et al.* (1991a) USA	6 nursing students	quasi	48%	4.0

Garg et al. (1991b) USA	6 nursing students	quasi	80%	4.5
Garg and Owen (1994) USA	57 nursing assistants	quasi	67%	4.5
Gingher et al. (1996) USA	52 nursing aides	quasi	78%	4.0
Kothiyal and Yven (2000) Australia	10 nurses	quasi	32%	4.0
Marras et al. (1999) USA	12 experienced and 5 inexperienced patient handlers	quasi	72%	5.0
Owen and Fragala (1999) USA	27 nurses	expt	59%	4.5
Roth et al. (1993) USA	23 nurses	quasi	57%	4.0
Ulin et al. (1997) USA	2 nurses	quasi	67%	5.0
Zhuang et al. (2000) USA	9 nursing assistants	quasi	54%	4.5
Zhuang et al. (1999) USA	9 nursing assistants	quasi	59%	4.5

☺☺☺ Moderate evidence from three studies for using mechanical (hoists) lifts for dependent (non-weight-bearing) patients

☺☺☺ Moderate evidence from five studies for using a walking belt with two carers for weight-bearing patients

☺☺☺ Moderate evidence from three studies for not using a walking belt with one carer for weight-bearing patients

☺☺☺ Moderate evidence from two studies that using a belt lifter (standing hoist) is preferable to manual methods

☺☺ Limited evidence from one study that sliding between a bed and a stretcher chair may be easier that using either a gait belt or a hoist

☺☺ Limited evidence from one study that using one or two handling slings with two carers is preferable to no slings

☹☹ Limited evidence from one study that using a gantry hoist is preferable to mobile hoists for bed–chair transfers

☺☺ Limited evidence from one study that a patient roller should be used for lateral transfers between bed and trolley

1   a walking harness attached to an overhead hoist to mobilise the patient on a
       treadmill; and
2   a standing hoist.

The author found that the walking hoist was fully supportive for collapsing or
overbalancing patients and could be used to secure and support a patient while
they were being positioned in a standing frame. She suggested that the standing
hoist could be used:

1   with patients who could support a limited amount of their own weight; and
2   to reinforce a sitting-to-standing pattern.

Khalil et al. (1987)

This study aimed to calculate the biomechanical stresses incurred on a nurse's
lower back while lifting a patient:

1   sitting up in bed from supine;
2   standing from sitting on the edge of the bed; and
3   standing up from a chair.

The authors calculated the force on the erector spinae and reactive force on L5/S1
and found that standing from a chair gave most load to nurses. However sitting
from lying supine gave the most reactive force at L5/S1.

Robertson et al. (1993)

The ability of kinesiotherapists to transfer patients from a wheelchair to a
standing frame was investigated. The authors measured the peak force, average
force, using a 2D biomechanical model and NIOSH equation to evaluate data.
The results showed that transferring patients weighing less than 16.9 kg could be
fairly safe, but that most female kinesiotherapists would be limited in personal
strength from lifting patients with body weights of more than 32 kg. The authors
suggested that a stooped posture would provide an improved lifting method with
respect to the action and maximal permissible NIOSH limits.

Ruszala (2001)

This M.Sc. dissertation evaluated four different types of equipment used in sit-to-
stand activities with patients during physiotherapy treatment programmes. The
outcome measures included RPE, REBA, BPDS, time for task and visual analogue
scales to collect data on ease of use, stability and effectiveness of task.

The findings split the equipment into two phases of rehabilitation:

Early rehabilitation:

1 hoist with walking harness;
2 standing hoist.

Functional activities:

1 chair lifter; and
2 patient turner (sit-stand-turn).

Ruszala found no significant difference between all four equipment types except for the time to carry out the task.

Summary of evidence

Author and location	Subjects	Study type	QR	PR
Busse (2000) UK	physiotherapists (n = ?)	PO	PO	3.5
Khalil et al. (1987) USA	2 nurses	quasi	7%	3.5
Robertson et al. (1993) USA	27 kinesiotherapists	quasi	71%	3.0
Ruszala (2001) UK	10 physiotherapists	expt	78%	5.0

☺☺ Limited evidence from one study that transferring patients weighing less than 16.9 kg might be safe

☺☺ Limited evidence from one study that a hoist with walking harness and a standing hoist are suitable for early rehabilitation, whereas a chair lifter and a patient turner (sit–stand–turn) are more suitable for functional activities

4.3 TRANSFERS IN STANDING

No literature was found to support the professional guidelines which recommend the techniques and equipment in Figure 6.

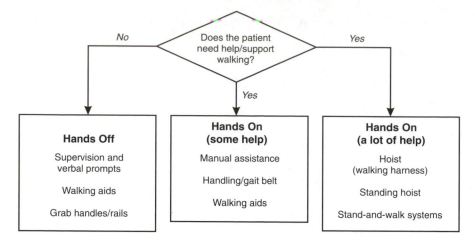

Figure 6 Transfers in standing

Suggestions from professional guidelines (not exhaustive)

☹   No literature was found to support the professional guidelines

CHAPTER 5

CARING TASKS

5.1 CARING TASKS FOR PATIENTS IN A LYING POSITION

5.1.1 Care and repositioning in lying

Ten papers are reviewed in this section to look at tasks carried out when the patient is lying down. These include hygiene tasks which might include turning or rolling, or repositioning in bed. The technique for the use of a piqué is suggested in two papers and the use a drawsheet for similar tasks in a further high-quality paper. Height-adjustable equipment was advocated in one high-quality study giving limited evidence. No research was found on the use of many of the equipment options recommended in professional guidelines (Figure 7).

Dolan and Adams (1998)

This study describes an evaluation of the effectiveness of various assistive aids and hoists in reducing the peak bending and compressive stresses acting on the lumbar spine. There were five tasks and three conditions: for this section the data for the task of turning in bed are presented. Four different techniques to achieve this task were tested:

1 log roll followed by manual slide;
2 turning device;
3 log roll followed by assisted slide with full-length transfer sheet with drawsheet; and
4 hoist.

Spinal compression was measured with EMG of the back muscles (with allowance for muscle length and contraction velocity). Spinal bending was measured as spinal curvature using electromagnetic motion analysis device over L5/S1.

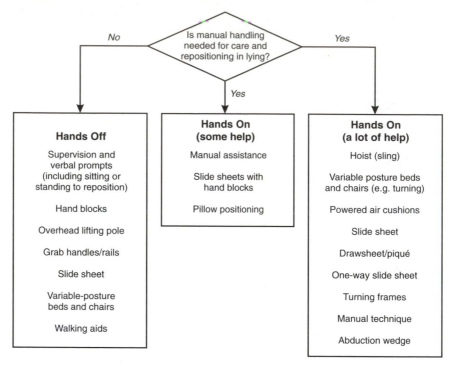

Figure 7 Care and repositioning in lying (including turning and rolling)
Suggestions from professional guidelines (not exhaustive)

The study found that sliding tasks tended to mimic manual tasks, except with the use of the turning device. The time taken was substantially increased when using the aids; however there was no significant difference in the time-dependent compression and flexion so they suggested that aids might take longer but are not necessarily more harmful. The various aids significantly reduced the peak and time-dependent loading of the lumbar spine but only by a modest amount. The effectiveness of the hoist only reduced peak compression loading by 5–23 per cent as it required nurses to adopt awkward stooped postures while securing and positioning the patient in the hoist.

Fourie (1992)

The purpose of this study was to demonstrate an improvement in the experimental group with respect to independent bridging and to reasonably infer that the mechanical advantage of pillow positioning was the cause of the improvement. A diagram was placed above the patient's bed with respect to the pillow positioning and the commands to be given to the patient (raise head and shoulders using the lifting pole in order to slide two pillows in lengthways; raise head to insert one pillow; release lifting pole and bridge to insert the bed pan).

The effect was measured by monitoring the number of days taken to achieve independent bridging. The study confirmed that this pillow positioning facilitates the functional use of the hip muscles with respect to the use of a bed pan.

Gagnon et al. (1987) and Gagnon and Lortie (1987)

This study used a detailed biomechanical analysis to look at the task of turning patients in bed using a 'piqué' (waterproof, padded sheet under patient), with six variations in the technique:

1   horizontal versus vertical pulling;
2   slow versus rapid;
3   leg position, symmetrical versus asymmetrical;
4   knee on bed or not;
5   low/high bed; and
6   free (manual) task.

Data were collected using a biomechanical dynamic model (eleven segments); EMG; and subjective rating of the task difficulty.

The findings indicated the preferred options for: horizontal pulling; rapid execution; knee on the bed; high bed. There was no preference with respect to leg position. The free (manual) task was perceived to be less strenuous but it was suggested that this might be due to experience resulting in a more efficient way of working.

The recommendations from the biomechanical evaluation suggest that the action of pulling and turning a patient in bed with a piqué should be accomplished with the forces being exerted in the vertical direction with the bed in a high (hip-level) position and rapid motion depending on the patient's condition. Knee support and leg position did not affect internal forces to any significant degree.

Gagnon et al. (1988a)

This study looked at pulling and/or turning patients across the bed using a piqué. The tasks were filmed for dynamic sequential analysis with a model of the spine to estimate spinal loadings; EMG for six specific muscles of the trunk, shoulder and elbow; three force platforms were used for both feet and one knee; total work requirements were evaluated using internal and external work, energy transfers, and the relative contribution of body segments to the work production.

The authors found that when the movement was interrupted with a pause to avoid sudden directional changes there were advantages related to: decrease in movement amplitude (hip movement); decrease on forces exerted on the piqué; significant decrease in the maximal activities on biceps. The resultant recommendation was that the use of a piqué for sliding should be taught with a pause to avoid sudden directional changes.

Gagnon et al. (1988b)

This paper described a preliminary study to explore the use of different design piqués to carry out the task of repositioning a patient from the centre to the side of the bed. Data were collected with video cameras and force platforms to carry out a detailed biomechanical analysis.

The results found no significant effect between the three different piqués; however, it was found that the method of carring out the handling task was greatly influenced by practice.

The authors recommended that the principles governing the teaching of patient handling needed to be reviewed, especially relating to the transfer of body weight and amplitude of segment movement.

Knibbe and Knibbe (1995)

This laboratory study measured the actual load on the musculoskeletal system of four nurses when washing, showering and bathing three patients using seven equipment options:

1   fixed-height bath;
2   fixed-height shower trolley;
3   fixed-height shower chair;
4   High–low bed (bed bath);
5   High–low bath;
6   High–low shower trolley; and
7   High–low shower chair.

OWAS and the time taken were used as outcome measures.

The findings showed that height-adjustable equipment gave rise to less physical stress than other equipment. The most harmful piece of equipment tested was the fixed-height shower chair. The study also showed that individual differences and preferences between nurses affect postural stress and time taken. Patient factors did not appear to have an effect, although real patients were not used.

Lindbeck and Engkvist (1993)

This study looked at the two tasks of:

1   turning a patient in bed; and
2   moving a patient up using a drawsheet and a friction-reducing plastic sheet.

Two techniques were used for each task:

Up in bed:

(a)   using one hand under the shoulder and one hand pulling on the drawsheet; and

(b)   two hands pulling on the drawsheet.

Turning:

(a)   high bed; and
(b)   low bed.

The outcome measures were: a 2D eleven-segment biomechanical model; a force plate for ground reaction force to estimate L5/S1 resultant force; video recordings of movement, rated perceived exertion.

The authors found that moving the patient up in bed required lower forces on the feet and hands than turning for both turning conditions (bed heights). Suggested explanations included that two carers could contribute equally to the task, whereas the different heights resulted in one carer exerting more force.

Marras et al. (1999)

This study aimed to identify the nature and range of low-back spinal forces and risk of low-back disorder associated with the various patient-handling tasks and techniques. This section includes the task of repositioning a patient in bed using the four following techniques:

1   one-carer hook and toss;
2   two-carer hook and toss;
3   two-carer drawsheet; and
4   two-carer thigh/shoulder lift.

Outcome measures included an EMG-assisted biomechanical model; LMM; and bipolar electrodes at the ten major trunk muscle sites.

The authors found that the one-carer hook-and-toss method (1) resulted in the highest low-back risk values. The best method to reposition in the bed was the drawsheet method with two carers (3). None of the transfers was considered hazardous for use in a hospital setting for either one or two carers. Both the biomechanical model and EMG indicated that none of the repositioning techniques was totally safe.

MDA (1997)

This study described a product evaluation of sixteen different handling products for moving dependent people in bed. The product types included:

1   sliding sheets;
2   short, low-friction rollers;
3   long, low-friction rollers; and
4   handling devices.

The products were allocated on a random basis and left with the carers for a period of one week. The outcome data were collected using a questionnaire and interview.

The authors found that short low-friction rollers were favoured over the other groups for moving people in bed. Named products were recommended for each group.

Summary of evidence

Author and location	Subjects	Study type	QR	PR
Dolan and Adams (1998) UK	25 female nurses	quasi	48%	5.0
Fourie (1992) South Africa	80 patients	expt	85%	5.0
Gagnon et al. (1987) Canada	15 female nursing aides	quasi	57%	4.0
Gagnon and Lortie (1987) Canada	15 female nursing aides	quasi	35%	3.5
Gagnon et al. (1988a) Canada	6 female subjects (no nursing experience)	quasi	44%	4.0
Gagnon et al. (1988b) Canada	2 female subjects (non nurses)	expt	63%	4.0
Knibbe and Knibbe (1995) Netherlands	4 nurses	quasi	56%	4.5
Lindbeck and Engkvist (1993) Sweden	12 physiotherapists	quasi	52%	4.0
Marras et al. (1999) USA	17 subjects, 12 experienced and 5 inexperienced	quasi	72%	5.0
MDA (1997) UK	57 carers from acute, community and private homes	quasi	77%	4.0

☺☺☺ Moderate evidence from two studies for the method of using a piqué (waterproof padded sheet) for turning a patient

☺☺   Limited evidence from one study that appropriate pillow positioning facilitates independent bridging

☺☺   Limited evidence from one study that using adjustable-height equipment for bathing is less physically stressful for carers

☺☺   Limited evidence from one study that the task of turning in bed may be more difficult than moving a patient up in bed

☺☺   Limited evidence from one study that using a drawsheet with two carers is less biomechanically stressful that other manual options

5.1.2   Repositioning in bed after hip surgery

This section looks at the evidence for moving patients in bed after total hip replacement (THR) surgery. The four included studies have all investigated this question from the perspective of the patients' safety rather than that of the carer. As all the studies addressed the same research question their findings are combined to give a limited-evidence-level statement.

King (1994)

This study described the results of a questionnaire survey of orthopaedic surgeons asking how patients could be moved post-THR to change from lifting-only practice. All the surgeons agreed that patients could be rolled, with the hip in a neutral position, rather than lifted (as most dislocations are due to the surgeon's procedure and not to patient positioning).

   The recommendation was to roll post-THR patients.

Love (1986)

This study gave a professional opinion based on a narrative literature review with respect to post-operative regimes for THR looking at three moving and handling options:

1   rolling patients onto side;
2   lifting with a lifting pole; and
3   orthodox lift.

Love's opinion was that the lifting pole was rarely used satisfactorily for nursing-care tasks as the patients tended to have reduced strength and endurance for a prolonged lift and often resulted in nurses giving assistance via a static orthodox lift.

   Love suggested that the preferred option should be rolling using an abduction pillow.

Love (1994)

This study looked at rolling and lifting post-THR. Love discussed alternative methods of rolling patients especially if a lifting pole was not used. The author suggested that a pelvic lift (with a carer at each side of the bed and hands grasped under the patient) was unsafe.

Love recommended that patients should be rolled.

Overd (1992)

This survey was carried out by postal questionnaire to look at current nursing practices in the positioning of patients following THR surgery. Thirty-seven wards (trauma, orthopaedic and trauma/orthopaedic combined) in nine hospitals were surveyed. Lifting was more commonly found on the orthopaedic and combined wards (80 per cent), whereas the trauma wards used rolling (to both sides). The study found that the orthopaedic wards consulted surgeons for advice and that the resultant practices were based on the surgeons' preference whereas the trauma wards made their own decisions.

The study concluded that there was a lack of reliable evidence for 'lift only' regimes so recommended that nurses should question this practice.

Summary of evidence

Author and location	Subjects	Study type	QR	PR
King (1994) UK	7 orthopaedic surgeons	survey	25%	3.0
Love (1986) UK	—	PO	PO	4.5
Love (1994) UK	—	PO	PO	3.5
Overd (1992) UK	32 wards	survey	41%	2.0

☺   Limited evidence for rolling THR patients rather than lifting

5.2 CARING TASKS FOR PATIENTS IN A SITTING POSITION

The six studies in this section look at tasks that take place in a sitting position. This includes repositioning a patient in a chair, and hygiene tasks which are

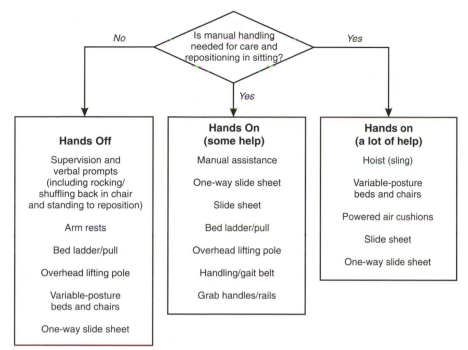

Figure 8 Care and repositioning in sitting
Suggestions from professional guidelines (not exhaustive)

carried out with the patient in a chair, wheelchair, commode or shower chair. Limited evidence from a single study suggests that most of the manual techniques investigated were potentially harmful. Additional findings suggest that equipment for hygiene tasks should be height-adjustable; a ramped wheelchair scale should be used to weigh dependent patients; and that repositioning a dependent patient in a wheelchair should be carried out with mechanical equipment.

Bruno and Davis (1997)

This paper described the evaluation of a standard hospital patient-transit wheelchair and proposed recommendations to maximise patient comfort and attendant ease of use. Difficulties were identified with catheter bags, brakes, chair-folding mechanisms, pillows and blankets. They produced a prototype design to address some of these problems. No evaluation of this prototype was reported.

Gabbett (1998)

This M.Sc. dissertation looked at:

1   shoulder lift versus shoulder slide; and

2   shoulder slide versus a reverse slide (for moving a seated patient up the
       bed).

The task was evaluated using biomechanical analysis (ground reaction forces),
REBA, RPE, BPDS and patient comfort.

The author found that there was no significant difference for using either the
shoulder lift or shoulder slide and that both were high-risk activities with respect
to low-back injury. There was also no significant difference between using either
the shoulder slide or the reverse slide.

Knibbe and Knibbe (1995)

This laboratory study measured the actual load on the musculoskeletal system of
four nurses when washing, showering and bathing three patients using seven
equipment options. OWAS and the time taken were used as outcome measures.

The findings showed that height-adjustable equipment gave rise to less physical stress than other equipment. The most harmful piece of equipment tested was
the fixed-height shower chair. The study also showed that individual differences
and preferences between nurses affect postural stress and time taken. Patient
factors did not appear to have an effect, although real patients were not used.

Owen and Garg (1994)

This study looked at the task of weighing a patient with three options for
achieving the task:

1   hook and toss with two carers from wheelchair on weighing-scale chair;
2   hoist with scales; and
3   wheelchair with ramp and platform.

The outcome measures included BPDS (with a ten-point scale), patient rating of
comfort, patient rating of security of posture, postural analysis using 3D static
biomechanical model (video), and pushing forces by post-hoc simulation with
hand force dynamometer.

The authors found that the manual option (1) was the most stressful,
followed by the hoist (2) and finally the wheelchair ramp (3) was the least
stressful, fastest and considered to be secure and comfortable.

Petzäll (1996)

This study aimed to work out a knowledge basis to specify heights of step obstacles possible to traverse with a manual wheelchair manoeuvred by an attendant
using two types of wheelchairs and two weights of patient:

1   a large front wheelchair pulled backwards; and

2   a large back wheelchair, pushed/tilted forwards.

The authors found that the same technique was used by all subjects (pushed/tilted forwards). The least demanding was the large back wheelchair, pushing forwards. A higher step resulted in increased difficulty – maximum 50 mm (or 100 mm if there was enough room to manoeuvre the wheelchair).

Varcin-Coad and Barrett (1998)

This study looked at three techniques for manually repositioning a slumped patient in a wheelchair:

1   unassisted lift with a through-arm grip;
2   vertically-assisted lift, with second person applying pressure upward on the knees; and
3   horizontally-assisted lift, through-arm, with the second person applying pressure horizontally on the knees.

Static biomechanical modelling was used to estimate L5/S1 compressive and shear forces acting on the spine of the carer behind the wheelchair.

For all techniques the L5/S1 compressive forces were found to be in excess of the back compression design limit. Technique 3 was the least stressful followed in order by Techniques 1 and 2. The recommendation was that mechanical equipment should be used for this task; if this was unavailable then the second carer applying a horizontal force on the knees resulted in lower stress for the carer positioned behind the wheelchair.

Summary of evidence

Author and location	Subjects	Study type	QR	PR
Bruno and Davis (1997) USA	30 staff at 5 hospitals and nursing homes	survey	7%	2.5
Gabbett (1998) UK	57 student nurses	expt	63%	4.5
Knibbe and Knibbe (1995) Netherlands	4 nurses	quasi	56%	4.5
Owen and Garg (1994) USA	6 female nursing students	quasi	50%	4.0
Petzäll (1996) Sweden	20 subjects (no detail)	quasi	48%	4.0

Varcin-Coad and Barrett (1998) Australia	16 female subjects (no detail)	quasi	65%	4.0

☺☺ Limited evidence from one study that shoulder lifts, shoulder slides or reverse slides are equally high-risk techniques for repositioning a sitting patient on a bed

☺☺ Limited evidence from one study that using adjustable-height equipment for bathing is less physically stressful for carers

☺☺ Limited evidence from one study that weighing a dependent patient should be done using a ramped wheelchair weigh scale

☺☺ Limited evidence from one study that manual repositioning a slumped patient in a wheelchair should be done with mechanical equipment

CHAPTER 6

SPECIALIST AREAS

The specialist areas of clinical practice covered in this chapter include the ambulance sector, operating theatres, rehabilitation, community and midwifery. We had hoped to also include a section on paediatrics but no research was found in the search.

6.1 AMBULANCE

This section reviews the available evidence on patient handling in ambulance work. The studies have been grouped into two subsections looking at:

1 the level of risk to ambulance personnel from performing patient-handling tasks; and
2 specialist equipment.

6.1.1 Level of risk to ambulance personnel from performing patient-handling tasks

Seven studies are reported which looked at the level of risk to ambulance personnel when carrying out manual handling tasks. The risks were greatest when patient handling tasks were being carried out, tending to result in harmful working postures, in particular over-reaching/over-stretching. Three of the studies had a QR of over 50 per cent so this evidence has been given a moderate rating.

Collins (1998)

This study measured the effect of using a back belt (worn by the carer) with an LMM for a range of ambulance tasks:

1 stretcher tasks;

2   transporting carry-chairs up/down stairs;
3   loading patients on carry-chairs on/off ambulances;
4   transferring from carry-chair to stretcher; and
5   transferring patients from one interface to another.

Results showed that the use of a back belt gave an overall reduction of all the measured risk factors, especially average rotational velocity, maximal sagittal flexion, and maximal side-bending velocity. The conclusion recommended the use of back belts for ambulance work.

Collins (1994)

This study assessed two tasks using the LMM:

1   lifting or carrying stretchers; and
2   carrying chairs.

The author found that 45 per cent of the assessments fell within the 40–50 per cent probability for low-friction discomfort, 45 per cent within 50–60 per cent and 10 per cent within 60–70 per cent (very high risk). No specific recommendations were given other than the comment that ambulance work would seem to be risky and that the design of carry-chairs has remained the same for thirty-five years.

Doormaal et al. (1995)

This study looked at the extent to which:

1   the working postures;
2   specific tasks and activities constituted a physical load for the musculo-skeletal system; and
3   ambulance assistants perceived their load.

These questions were investigated using:

●   OWAS;
●   work and health questionnaire for perceived work load (WHQ); and
●   ARB5 biomechanical model.

The authors found that 16–29 per cent of the working postures during a shift were spent in harmful postures, including static and short-duration, maximal-exertion lifting tasks and often having to work in uncomfortable positions. However they also commented that lifting techniques differed widely. Their recommendations included specific training and a reduction in lifting by using hospital under-frames and encouraging patient self help (independence) as well as design improvements for seating in the patient compartment (in ambulance).

Furber et al. (1997)

In order to identify associated factors, 1,039 work-related injuries were reviewed over a two-year period for ambulance staff to identify associated factors.

The authors found that 58 per cent of injuries involved the patient, with 41 per cent of injuries occurring while using some form of mechanical aid, of which 35 per cent involved a stretcher. Forty-nine per cent of injuries occurred at a private residence compared with 19 per cent in a hospital. The most common event was overexertion/overreaching (80 per cent). They recommended a review of stretcher design.

Massad et al. (2000)

This paper described a two-part study. The first part used a one-day training session to investigate staff perceptions of:

1   bed-to-ambulance trolley transfer (a) sitting and (b) lying;
2   lateral slide board techniques;
3   design changes to ambulance vehicle (height for loading); stretcher; stretcher-activating devices and brakes.

The authors reported the perception as being highly successful for training with respect to two lateral transfer techniques in sitting and lying.

The second part of the study involved analysing 139 accidents to identify the highest-risk actions. These were found to be:

1   the transportation of equipment on which patients were sitting or lying in staircases, elevators or in the street (24 per cent of accidents);
2   patient handling and transfers (14 per cent); and
3   loading and unloading of stretcher (with the patient) in/out of ambulance (12 per cent).

McGill et al. (1990)

This paper looked at the low-back demands on ambulance attendants for the following tasks with two attendants:

1   lifting a patient from the floor without equipment;
2   carrying a patient;
3   carrying a patient upstairs in a cot (stretcher);
4   lifting a patient in a clamshell (scoop) stretcher from the floor;
5   lifting a cot and patient from the ground into an ambulance;
6   lifting a patient on a spine board from a slope;
7   lifting a patient out of a chair; and
8   lifting a chair (plastic seat pan) with a patient sitting in it;

and the following two tasks with one attendant:

9   lifting a patient from a bed using a curl lift (placement of arms underneath a supine patient and hug to body); and
10   rolling a patient off a couch.

A video recording was used for a biomechanical analysis.

The authors found that most of the tasks generated compressive forces on the lumbar joints which exceeded the maximum permissible limit (NIOSH). Taller staff experienced greater loads on the spine due to difficulties in positioning their feet under the load. The most demanding tasks involved lifting a patient from the ground. They recommended:

1   additional handles on the clamshell stretcher; and
2   the development of a lighter cot.

Torma-Krajewski (1987)

The author carried out a study to identify and evaluate manual-handling tasks performed by paramedics (and other health-care workers). She collected data using job analysis (description from supervisor, weight limits, availability of equipment and assistance) and biomechanical analysis with grading using NIOSH guidelines (assuming all lifts were in sagittal place and carried out in a slow, symmetrical manner with a static component at the start and end of the lift).

The results of the fourteen paramedic tasks found that nine were in Category 3 (exceeding maximum permissible load (NIOSH), only possible by 1 per cent of women and 25 per cent of men):

- lifting patient onto ground stretcher (arm–leg);
- lifting patient from stretcher to bed (side);
- lifting round stretcher into ambulance;
- removing stretcher from ambulance (end);
- removing ground stretcher from ambulance (side);
- raising stretcher (low to high);
- carrying stretcher down steps; and
- using a backboard to lift patient.

One task was in Category 2 (possible by 75 per cent of women and 99 per cent of men):

- lifting patient onto ground stretcher (straight).

The author concluded that lifting tasks for paramedics were very stressful due to the high weights and large horizontal distances of the hands.

Summary of evidence

Author and location	Subjects	Study type	QR	PR
Collins (1998) UK	2 ambulance personnel	quasi	19%	3.0
Collins (1994) UK	Ambulance personnel (n = ?)	quasi	4%	2.0
Doormaal et al. (1995) Netherlands	30 ambulance assistants (15 nurses, 15 drivers)	x-sect.	64%	3.5
Furber et al. (1997) Australia	1,163 ambulance personnel	survey	66%	4.0
Massad et al. (2000) Canada	215 ambulance technicians	survey	55%	3.5
McGill et al. (1990) Canada	4 subjects	x-sect.	32%	3.5
Torma-Krajewski (1987) USA	Paramedics (n = ?)	x-sect.	43%	2.5

☺☺☺ Moderate evidence from three studies that ambulance work can result in harmful working postures, with the highest-risk tasks involving transportation of patients on equipment

6.1.2   Specialist equipment: stretcher carrying/loading

Four studies are included which describe the use of stretchers, both for carrying and loading into an ambulance. As these are single studies only a limited evidence rating has been given.

Knapik et al. (2000)

This study evaluated four ways of carrying stretchers in field conditions (military medical):

1   by hand;
2   using cross-shoulder straps;
3   using a harness to shift the load between hip and shoulder; and
4   using load carriage equipment, hip-bearing via a belt clip.

The outcome measures used for data collection included heart rate, oxygen uptake, RPE, time to fatigue, subjective rating for pain, soreness and discomfort.

The authors found that the carrying times were longest for Options 3 and 4. The hand carriage, Option 1, resulted in significantly more cardiorespiratory stress than the other options. The upper-body RPE rating was lower in Options 3 (hip/shoulder) and 4 (hip-bearing), and these were also preferred for comfort, ease of use and stability.

Lavender et al. (2000a)

This study analysed five tasks used for emergency evacuation:

1 transferring a patient from bed to stretcher using a bed sheet;
2 transferring a patient from stretcher to hospital gurney (trolley) using a bed sheet;
3 lifting and transporting a patient down the stairs and around a landing using a back board;
4 transporting a patient down a straight set of stairs using a stretcher; and
5 transporting a patient down the stairs and around a landing using a stair-chair.

Data were collected using an LMM and two biomechanical models.

The authors found that there were strength limitations with 71 per cent of the population able to carry out Task 1; 86 per cent Task 2, and 53 per cent Task 3. All the activities showed a high level of risk. The authors recommended engineering changes to the equipment regularly used by emergency-rescue personnel.

Lavender et al. (2000b)

This paper described the same study as Lavender *et al.* (2000a) but reported the working postures encountered in the listed tasks. Postures were analysed using an LMM.

The authors found that a variety of different methods was used for each task, with the stretcher-to-gurney transfer being the least strenuous. They recommended that:

1 a lower level of postural risk was recorded for Task 1 if the paramedic stood at the side of the bed rather than with their knee on the bed; and
2 a low-friction interface (bridging) board reduced the friction force for all lateral transfers.

Stevenson (1995)

Using observations over ten shifts (including three night shifts), this study evaluated different ambulance tasks:

1 loading/unloading onto the raised/lowered stretcher;
2 lifting the stretcher; and
3 loading/unloading the stretcher into/out of the ambulance.

The author found that there was an average of 11.9 patient transfers per shift; with 5.5 full weight lifts per shift. The lifts included: fore and aft lift; flat (total weight-bearing lift); lift on stretcher; carry sheet; chair lift (no chair); spine board. The easy-load style stretcher weighed 46 kg (including bedding) and was available at two heights (low and high). Neonatal retrieval units on top of the stretcher resulted in additional weight of 145 kg. He recommended lifting one end of the stretcher at a time (if the patient's condition does not preclude it) so that the load be shared between two ambulance officers. Design recommendations for stretchers included extending handles and intermediate-height positions.

Summary of evidence

Author and location	Subjects	Study type	QR	PR
Knapik et al. (2000) USA	11 soldiers	quasi	57%	4.5
Lavender et al. (2000a) USA	20 paramedics/fire fighters	quasi	61%	5.0
Lavender et al. (2000b) USA	20 paramedics/fire fighters	x-sect.	59%	4.5
Stevenson (1995) Australia	ambulance officers (n = ?)	x-sect.	43%	3.5

☺☺ Limited evidence that stretcher bearing could be made safer by bearing some of the weight through the hip; by using two staff to lift each end; and by reducing the vertical height lifts (lower tail gate)

6.2 THEATRES

This section presents five studies which looked at different aspects of patient handling in theatres. Two studies collected data using observations and a survey and concluded that transfers were only carried out with two staff even when more were available. Both studies also found that most patient transfers were carried out using poles and canvas. Two studies suggested a wider drawsheet/canvas for lateral transfers with a sliding aid. Other studies confirmed that equipment, in particular mechanical equipment, was not generally used. However the quality ratings were low so the evidence statement has been graded as 'limited'.

Coleman and Brooke (1999)

An observational survey was described which looked at the techniques used to transfers patients to/from the operating table – who was involved and the general hazards. Data were collected using observation, a chronological record of events and structured interviews.

The authors found that thirty out of thirty-six transfers were carried out with poles and canvas and of these 75 per cent were obstructed by anaesthetic machines, resulting in lateral flexion. Forty-four per cent of transfers only involved two staff, even when more were available. They concluded by recommending the use of a wider canvas.

Garb and Dockery (1995)

This study described an ergonomic assessment and resultant implementation of recommendations over an eighteen-month period. The assessment included:

1   walk-through;
2   detailed observation of five surgical procedures;
3   staff interviews;
4   measurement of equipment (dimensions, force to use, etc.); and
5   postural analysis.

Five recommendations were implemented of which one related to manual handling: using four people with a low-friction sliding board and wider draw-sheet for an operating table–stretcher/bed transfer. The outcome measure recorded the number of back injuries. A 25 per cent reduction in operating-room injuries was recorded within the first six months. However eighteen months after the intervention they reported that the injury rate was increasing.

Luntley et al. (1995)

This survey examined the pattern of manual handling of patients in the operating theatre and the level of knowledge of anaesthetists about the manual-handling operations regulations. The outcome measures included:

1   number of staff performing manoeuvre;
2   method used;
3   weight of patient; and
4   twisting/awkward postures.

The authors found that 96 per cent of the transfers were performed by two staff even when more staff were available. Sixteen of the twenty-two anaesthetists (73 per cent) questioned regularly lifted patients although none had received any moving and handling training. The equipment used was found to be poles and canvas (91 per cent) and lateral transfer boards (9 per cent).

MacKenzie et al. (1997)

This study described the development of a limb-support system (support cuffs for nurses' wrists when holding patient limbs) for preparing a patient in theatres. The system aimed to reduce the cumulative strain from risks involving duration (2–10 minutes), poor posture (twisting and side flexion). The limb-support system is a ceiling-mounted, electrically-braked cable which has a constant force, spring-retraction system, operated by a control button worn on a nurse's index finger.

No formal evaluation was undertaken although positive comments were recorded during the development process.

McKellar and Shaw (1986)

This study explored the potential for using mechanised lifting in theatres through an informal survey of forty-eight theatres (two with hoists, eighteen with transfer systems). They discussed the use of mechanised lifting equipment in the context of the sophisticated equipment which is provided for anaesthesia/ventilation.

The study concluded that it was difficult to justify the lack of availability of mechanical systems in theatres to move 70-kg delicate products (human beings).

6.3   REHABILITATION

This section includes eight studies relating to patient transfers in rehabilitation. Five papers considered the use of equipment in rehabilitation, advocating the use of adjustable-height equipment. Standing hoists with walking harness are shown to be useful rehabilitation aids.

Billin (2001)

Two case studies were described with respect to manual handling in a neuro-disability environment. Both cases used mesh hoist slings which were described as being useful for patients with complex extensor patterns who tended to slide out of regular slings. This type of sling can be left in place under the patient.

Busse (2000)

This study looked at the use of hoists in rehabilitation using a functional impendence measure to assess the patient's initial dependency. Two types of hoist were used for the rehabilitation programme:

Summary of evidence

Author and location	Subjects	Study type	QR	PR
Coleman and Brooke (1999) UK	theatre staff (n = ?)	x-sect.	39%	3.5
Garb and Dockery (1995) USA	14 room surgical suite (theatre/OR staff)	quasi	56%	3.5
Luntley et al. (1995) UK	22 anaesthetists	survey	52%	4.0
MacKenzie et al. (1997) UK	theatre staff (n = ?)	PO	PO	4.5
McKellar and Shaw (1986) UK	theatre staff (n = ?)	PO	PO	3.5

☺☺   Limited evidence that many patient transfers in theatres will be carried out by only two staff even when more are available

☺☺   Limited evidence that poles and canvas are the most commonly used system of patient transfer in theatres

1   a walking harness attached to an overhead hoist to mobilise the patient on a treadmill; and

2   a standing hoist.

The author found that the walking hoist was fully supportive for collapsing or overbalancing patients and it could be used to secure and support a patient while they were being positioned in a standing frame. She suggested that the standing hoist could be used with patients who could support a limited amount of their own weight and to reinforce a sitting-to-standing pattern.

Fenety and Kumar (1991)

As part of a workplace survey this study looked at the manual handling found in a physiotherapy department. Patients were the most common load for lifting, with the most common tasks being:

1   assisting patients to stand;
2   assisting sitting–sliding transfers;
3   repositioning in wheelchairs; and
4   assisting supine patients to roll over.

The working postures during patient transfers were nearly always constrained by either equipment (e.g. wheelchairs) or patient factors (e.g. poor balance or safety). Hidden strains occurred when physiotherapists were kneeling on raised mats, with approximately a third of the treatment time spent in a stooped posture.

The authors concluded by recommending that adjustable-height beds/mats should be used for treatment.

Hignett (2001a)

This qualitative study, set in an acute hospital, reported a manual-handling risk-assessment process with occupational therapists and subsequent proposed intervention programme. A large number of risks assessments were rationalised into three themes:

1   treatment handling – to be addressed by the development of local standards and criteria for practice;
2   interagency communication – joint problem solving sessions were held for physiotherapists and occupational therapists to explore their respective roles and treatment-handling issues; and
3   non-hospital property – looked at the complexity of the provision of a safe working environment by the property owner.

It was suggested that some of the risks should be managed through negotiation within the service contract. The recommendations suggested that a residual level of unpredictability would always be underlying for manual handling in occupational therapy which needed further exploration.

Jackson and Liles (1994)

This study analysed the working postures, in particular transfer techniques, of physiotherapy students using OWAS. No hoists were used and the physiotherapy students made minimal analysis of avoidable risks with respect to altering the task or environment before attempting a transfer.

The result was that very few of the observed transfers were acceptable in practice. More hazardous postures were observed in neurological rehabilitation settings (mostly standing transfers, action category 3–4) than in out-patient physiotherapy.

Robertson et al. (1993)

This study looked at the ability of kinesiotherapists to transfer patients from a wheelchair to a standing frame. Data were collected on the peak force and average force using 2D biomechanical model, and the NIOSH equation.

The authors found that transferring patients weighing less than 16.9 kg could be fairly safe. Most female kinesiotherapists would be limited in personal strength from lifting patients with body weights of more than 32 kg. The recommendation was that a stooped posture would provide an improved lifting method with respect to the action and maximal permissible NIOSH limits.

Ruszala (2001)

This M.Sc. dissertation evaluated four different types of equipment used in sit-to-stand activities with patients during physiotherapy treatment programmes. The outcome measures included RPE, REBA, BPDS, time for task and visual analogue scales to collect data on ease of use, stability and effectiveness of task.

The findings split the equipment into two phases of rehabilitation.

Early rehabilitation:

1   hoist with walking harness; and
2   standing hoist.

Functional activities:

1   chair lifter; and
2   patient turner (sit–stand–turn).

The author found no significant difference between all four equipment types except for the time taken to carry out the task.

Sparkes (2001)

This study examined and discussed the problems with an assisted transfer (pivot) used in the process of neurological rehabilitation by the physiotherapy treatment approaches described by Bobath and Carr and Shepherd. The author suggested that neither of the approaches had demonstrated their effectiveness or outcome measures in the light of MHOR regulations.

6.4   COMMUNITY/HOME CARE

This section brings together the available research on patient handling tasks (6.4.1), equipment (6.4.2) and interventions (6.4.3) for community and home-care nursing. This includes nursing and residential homes as well as domestic (private) homes.

Summary of evidence

Author and location	Subjects	Study type	QR	PR
Billin (2001) UK	2 female patients	case	23%	3.0
Busse (2000) UK	physiotherapists (n = ?)	PO	PO	3.5
Fenety and Kumar (1991) Canada	physiotherapy staff (n = ?)	survey	18%	3.0
Hignett (2001a) UK	12 occupational therapists	qual.	85%	5.0
Jackson and Liles (1994) UK	physiotherapy students	x-sect.	66%	4.0
Robertson et al (1993) USA	27 kinesiotherapists	quasi	71%	3.0
Ruszala (2001) UK	10 physiotherapists	expt	78%	5.0
Sparkes (2001) UK	—	PO	PO	4.0

☹☹ Limited evidence from one study that manual-handling risks for occupational therapists can be complex involving inter-agency issues for non-hospital property

☺☹ Limited evidence from one study that physiotherapy students adopt harmful postures when transferring patients, particularly during neurological rehabilitation

☺☺ Limited evidence from one study that a stooped posture may provide an improved lifting method for female kinesiotherapists to transfer patients from a wheelchair to a standing frame

☺☹ Limited evidence from one study that a hoist with a walking harness and a standing hoist are suitable for early rehabilitation, whereas a chair lifter and patient turner are more suitable for functional activities

6.4.1 Tasks

This section includes five studies, three of which suggest that manual handling difficulties may be associated with patients' beds. One good-quality study recommends that nurses should work in pairs.

Ballard (1994)

This survey of manual-handling activities by district nurses considered the impact of employment policy changes on workload and perceived effects of mental health.

The reported results identified difficulties in lifting patients due to poor access to the patient's bed frequently or sometimes (90 per cent).

Brulin et al. (2000)

This qualitative study aimed to gain a deeper understanding of the factors in the work environment of home-care personnel which were perceived as demanding or problematic.

It was found that the staff were highly affected by demanding psychosocial and physical working conditions, including time pressure and physically demanding tasks. The poor physical work environment was also found to be a factor.

Knibbe and Friele (1996)

This study looked at transfers in a community setting by asking nurses to ask if they could describe any moments they considered to be physically demanding.

The qualitative data were analysed thematically to give a hierarchy of frequency of occurrence. The authors found that the most demanding tasks were listed as bed transfers: bed actions (37 per cent); bed transfers (31 per cent); bed to wheelchair (22 per cent); bathing (static load, 23 per cent).

Lusted et al. (1996)

This study described different work practices with respect to neck and upper-limb symptoms in a residential-care centre for the developmentally disabled, with all the patients being wheelchair users. The work practices were investigated using observation, heart-rate monitors, RPE, local-discomfort ratings, and a record of the type of activity being performed (e.g. bathing, dressing, feeding) on a fifteen-minute checklist.

The authors found that most of the heavy physical work was carried out in the early part of the morning shift. Dressing and undressing patients was one of the most strenuous tasks and often resulted in wrist pain: it accounted for 12 per cent of time in the morning shift, and required considerable strength and static muscle work to separate and straighten the patients' limbs against the spastic muscles. Neck and upper-limb problems were more common in the unit where the nurses worked alone, with the RPE ratings being significantly higher compared with the unit where the nurses worked in pairs. They concluded by recommending that nursing staff should work in pairs.

Skarplik (1988)

This small survey reported about low-back pain and issues/practical advice for district/community nurses with respect to patient handling.

The issues identified included low beds, double beds, small bathrooms, soft mattresses, and crouching in a cramped environment.

Summary of evidence

Author and location	Subjects	Study type	QR	PR
Ballard (1994) UK	373 district nurses	survey	66%	4.0
Brulin et al. (2000) Sweden	8 home-care workers	qual.	73%	4.0
Knibbe and Friele (1996) Netherlands	355 community nurses	survey	77%	3.0
Lusted et al. (1996) Australia	10 nurses	x-sect.	66%	4.0
Skarplik (1988) UK	—	PO	PO	2.0

☺☺☺ Moderate evidence from three studies that manual-handling difficulties for community nursing are associated with patient beds

☺☺ Limited evidence from one study that nursing staff should work in pairs when caring for developmentally disabled patients

6.4.2 Equipment

The second section groups four studies which look at the use of equipment. There is only one high-quality study (limited evidence) which found that the introduction of hoists provided a solution for approximately 33 per cent of transfers in a nursing home. Another high-quality study (limited evidence) identified potential difficulties with introducing hoists into patient homes.

Conneeley (1998)

In the context of a wider study this qualitative paper explored patients' attitudes to being hoisted at home.

The author summarised by saying that the introduction of a hoist into a home was a complex issue. There needed to be consideration of the needs as perceived by the patient and the context of the whole environment (physical, social and psychological) for success.

Knibbe and Friele (1999)

This intervention included the provision of forty patient hoists being introduced over a twelve-month period in 139 nursing homes compared with 239 control nursing homes, with training, ergonomic assessment forms and lifting coordinators. The outcome measures included RPE, general epidemiological information and a specifically-designed recording tool (Log). The Log has eleven categories of nursing activity relating to patient transfer; three options of patient cooperation; number of carers involved; assistance from informal care; use of equipment; and patient weight.

The authors found that the twelve-month back pain prevalence was reduced significantly in the intervention group, whereas the control group showed no change. The Log showed a decrease in the exposure for wheelchair transfers, bed transfers, and showering (sitting). The conclusion was that hoists provided a solution for approximately 33 per cent of the total number of transfers. The intervention group had a reduction in transfers for both hoist (50 per cent) and non-hoist (35 per cent) transfers, with no change in the control group. At the end of the intervention all passive patients in the intervention group were lifted with a hoist (compared with 67 per cent at the start).

Menoni et al. (1999)

This paper reported a study which aimed to evaluate the level of risk from moving patients in both acute hospital wards and geriatric residences. The outcome measure used included:

1   the MAPO index of exposure to identify prevention and improvement measures;
2   ratio between cooperative and uncooperative patients to nursing personnel on three shifts;
3   evaluation of equipment for transferring patients;
4   wheelchair evaluation;
5   environment evaluation; and

6   training and information.

The authors found that residential homes showed a higher level of exposure (42 per cent of workers) to risk than most hospital wards (28 per cent). They suggested that the higher values were due to a severe shortage of hoists and minor aids, poor training and lack of information.

Proteau (2000)

This study described an evaluation of a training programme for home-care workers in Canada for two staff groups. The first group were Social Family Assistants (SFAs), where 80 per cent of tasks involved bathroom hygiene with problems of getting clients in/out of the tub.

It was found that equipment helped with wall mounts (grab rails); plastic stools to put the patient's feet on to wash and for SFAs to sit on at the same height; and hospital-style, adjustable-height beds. The second group were home-care nurses, where accidents included falls on stairs and problems with transporting equipment to/from the car. Improvements included a bag with a shoulder strap/back pack.

Summary of evidence

Author and location	Subjects	Study type	QR	PR
Conneeley (1998) UK	10 patients	qual.	92%	5.0
Knibbe and Friele (1999) Netherlands	378 home-care nurses	quasi	83%	5.0
Menoni et al. (1999) Italy	216 wards in 20 centres	x-sect.	57%	3.0
Proteau (2000) Canada	social family assistants (n = ?) home-care nurses (n = ?)	PO	PO	4.0

☺☺   Limited evidence from one study to support the use of hoists in nursing and residential homes

☺☺   Limited evidence from one study to identify potential difficulties with introducing hoists into patient homes

6.4.3   Interventions

The final section groups six intervention studies. All these studies used a multi-factor intervention (see Chapter 11, page 150), with most being based on risk assessment. The evidence-level statement is moderate: that using a multi-factor intervention reduces lost time due to back pain and biomechanical indices.

Alexander (1996)

This project evaluated a risk-management programme for community nurses with respect to the nursing manager's ability to implement the recommendations for risk reduction. The risk-reduction recommendations included provision of hoists, increasing staffing levels, addressing space constraints, tackling difficulties identified with both patients and carers (including sudden changes in clinical condition).

The author found that the managers perceived that an increased awareness through education would be the main factor in reducing sickness absence for back and neck pain whereas the staff believed that provision of equipment would be the main factor. A significant relationship was found with respect to implementation of risk reduction recommendations and reduction in sickness absence. It was found to be three times lower (9 per cent compared with 28 per cent) in the implementation group than the non-implementation group over the twelve-month period.

Best (1997)

This paper investigated the hypothesis that thirty-two hours' training in the manutention method of manual handling would decrease back strain and injuries in nurses working in geriatric care. The intervention was evaluated with:

1   postural analysis (OWAS);
2   a questionnaire about the frequency and severity of back pain;
3   RPE; and
4   nurses' perception of patient comfort and safety.

Over the twelve-month period no significant results were found for the postural analysis, RPE ratings or reported injuries, although all showed some improvement over the pre-intervention data.

Garg and Owen (1992)

This paper described a four-year ergonomic intervention in nursing homes which aimed to reduce back stress. In this paper stages 5 and 6 are described of the six-stage intervention:

1   determination of patient-handling tasks perceived to be most stressful by nursing aides (Owen and Garg, 1989);
2   ergonomic evaluation of the work performed by nursing assistants prior to the introduction of change (Carlson, 1989);
3   pilot study to identify and locate assistive devices, to establish criteria for their selection and perform preliminary trials (Owen and Garg, 1990);
4   laboratory study on patient-handling devices (Garg *et al.*, 1991a and b);
5   intervention of selected devices into nursing homes and the training of NAs to use them with patients;
6   post-intervention measurement of back-injury incidence and severity rates, acceptability rates, biomechanical task demands and perceived level of physical stress.

The following tasks were used for training: transfer bed–wheelchair; wheelchair–toilet; wheelchair–chairlift; in/out of bath tub; weighing patient. Hoists, walking belts with handles and a shower chair with removable foot pedals and arm supports were provided as additional equipment. The patients were classified as weight-bearing and dependent (use walking belt to transfer); dependent and non-weight-bearing (use hoist to transfer) and independent. The intervention was evaluated using acceptability rates (compliance with equipment assessed by observation); RPE; biomechanical evaluation; incidence of low-back pain; time for transfers; and number of NAs used in each transfer.

Overall the authors found that there was an 81–96 per cent acceptance for the devices; the biomechanical stresses were significantly reduced (below the NIOSH action limit); the RPE for hoist and walking belt was reported as very, very light and very light; the injury rates fell from 83 per 200,000 work hours lost to 47 per 200,000 work hours lost. The authors concluded by saying that a systematic and appropriate ergonomic intervention could significantly reduce physical stresses to NAs and therefore reduce the future risk of musculoskeletal injuries.

Nyran (1991)

This study aimed to measure the direct costs of implementing an intervention programme in relation to the costs of patient-handling-related injuries among nursing personnel in nursing homes. A training programme was used which included a two-day course (including ergonomic risk assessment) with a five-hour follow-up at six months. Actions from the risk assessments were implemented during the intervention including: purchase of hoists, variable-height beds; new wheelchairs with detachable arm/leg rests; and equipment maintenance. The intervention was evaluated using:

1   injury status eight months prior to the training, and eight months after;
2   lost-time claims from the compensation board; and
3   additional data from interviews with senior and middle managers before and after the training.

The results showed that there was a net saving of $57,440 (saving in lost-time injuries, including the cost of the training) in four out of the five nursing homes. The conclusion was that intensive training had some impact on the reduction in the number of workers' compensation board claims. The interviews suggested that there was a reduction in the severity of the cases.

Peers (1998)

This intervention used:

1   risk assessments;
2   individual bedside logos for correct method of transfer;
3   assessment of every resident before lift/transfer;
4   education programme; and
5   provision of sliding sheets for repositioning in bed.

The evaluation looked at lost time and the number of staff on decreased work-capacity.

Following the interventions there was a reduction in lost time and number of staff on modified duties.

Pohjonen et al. (1998)

This study described an investigation into the effects and feasibility of a twelve-month ergonomic intervention on work content and load in home-care work. Various ergonomic measures were included which were designed and implemented as part of a participatory approach based on team work and group problem-solving within the work unit. The interventions included

1   group problem-solving;
2   changing/redesigning the equipment used;
3   purchase of new equipment;
4   changing the methods for using equipment;
5   increasing the possibilities for regulating the work pace; and
6   discussing the goals of the work with the clients.

Work-site assessments included questionnaires (including Work Ability Index), work sampling study, work physiological measurements (heart-rate monitor) and postural analysis (OWAS).

The proportion of straight back positions increased significantly due to the intervention (from 59 to 75 per cent). Subjects were better able to utilise their own abilities and needs to adjust the work rate as a result of the intervention. The ergonomic measures improved both physical and mental work content and working conditions and prevented the decline of work ability in the intervention group. The conclusion was that participatory ergonomics was an effective and feasible way of reducing the work load and increasing the job satisfaction of ageing female home-care workers.

Summary of evidence

Author and location	Subjects	Study type	QR	PR
Alexander (1996) UK	42 community nurse managers, 93 community nurses	survey	50%	5.0
Best (1997) Australia	55 nursing and allied health staff at 3 nursing homes	quasi	70%	3.0
Garg and Owen (1992) USA	57 nursing assistants	quasi	63%	5.0
Nyran (1991) Canada	48 nurses	case	65%	4.0
Peers (1998) Canada	131 nursing home staff	quasi	37%	3.0
Pohjonen et al. (1998) Finland	70 home-care workers	expt	58%	4.5

☺☺☺   Moderate evidence from three studies that using multi-factor interventions, based on risk assessments, reduces lost time due to back pain

☺☺   Limited evidence from one study that manutention training has no effect on working postures, RPE or injury rates

6.5   MIDWIFERY

This section about midwifery is made up of four high-quality studies. The evidence shows that midwives perform different tasks from nurses and that changes in birthing postures can affect the risk of injury to midwives. Despite the high-quality rating of the studies all deal with different aspects of midwifery so the evidence levels are graded as 'limited'.

Hignett (1996a)

This paper described a qualitative exploratory study looking at the factors contributing to the high level of reported musculoskeletal injuries. Data were collected using focus groups, observation and individual interviews. The thematic analysis (using NUD*IST) resulted in sixty-eight codes. The following factors were identified: the handling of two loads (mother and baby);

relationship of midwife with mother (advocate), etc. Midwives have different tasks and patients to general nurses, e.g. assisting breast feeding and delivery.

Mulligan et al. (1988)

This study looked at the evacuation of neonatal babies from a nursery.
The authors recommended:

1   using cribs and pushing to evacuation point;
2   evacubabe aprons, with six pouches in an apron to carry a maximum of six babies; and
3   a backpack for evacuation of supplies, and for resuscitation equipment.

Thompson (2000)

This postural-analysis study looked at the working postures for midwives when assisting with current delivery positions. Data were collected with OWAS and REBA.
The study resulted in recommendations to modify positions to improve working postures for midwives as follows:

1   mother in long sitting with knees bent and abducted with a back support and the end off the delivery bed;
2   mother kneeling on the bed, facing head of bed, move mother to bottom of bed (take bed end off) and raise bed height;
3   mother standing and forward leaning (not kneeling) onto bed – midwife sitting or kneeling behind, centrally;
4   mother side lying with one leg supported – raise height of bed and put mother onto side of bed.

Waldenström and Gottvall (1991)

This randomised, controlled trial compared 294 women using a birthing stool or a semi-recumbent position in the second stage of labour. Outcome measures included obstetric outcome, infant outcome, mother's expectation recorded with a questionnaire, and midwife's opinion.
The results showed no difference between the two groups in obstetric outcome, but that the mothers using the birthing stool experienced less pain and were more satisfied with the position. However the midwives found the postures that they needed to assume with the birthing stool very awkward.

Summary of evidence

Author and location	Subjects	Study type	QR	PR
Hignett (1996a) UK	42 midwives	qual.	96%	5.0
Mulligan et al. (1988) USA	–	PO	PO	3.0
Thompson (2000) UK	4 midwifery areas (n = ?)	survey	57%	4.0
Waldenström and Gottvall (1991) Sweden	294 pregnant women	expt	93%	5.0

☺☺   Limited evidence from one study that midwives perform different tasks from nurses

☺☺   Limited evidence from one study that changes in birthing postures can reduce the risk of injury to midwives

☺☺   Limited evidence from one study that midwives find that assisting a mother on a birthing stool leads to awkward working postures

SECTION III

EQUIPMENT

CHAPTER 7

SMALL AIDS

This chapter brings together the available research on small aids. This includes such devices as sliding sheets, handling/gait belts (worn by the patient), lifting (back) belts (worn by the carer), handling slings, turntables, sliding boards, rope ladders, hand blocks, one-way glide sheets. Devices associated with beds such as lifting poles are included in Chapter 8 (Beds).

7.1 SLIDING SHEETS

Section 7.1 looks at the evidence from seven studies with respect to the use of sliding sheets. There is moderate evidence that double-thickness (roller or two separate) sliding sheets are preferable to single-thickness sliding sheets. Other evidence from this section is classed as limited as it is either based on single studies or poor-quality studies. These conclude that handles on sliding sheets do not alter the stress on the lower back and that short, low-friction roller sheets are the preferred option for moving people up in bed, as well as studies reporting comparative product evaluations which resulted in local purchasing recommendations.

Hignett (1999)

The subjects for this user trial of eighteen slide-sheets were professional back-care advisers. Four tasks were carried out with the various sheets:

1   sliding up the bed in a lying position;
2   sliding up the bed in a sitting position;
3   rolling; and
4   moving from sitting to lying.

A range of measurement criteria were applied to each piece of equipment to result in a final cumulative score.

Three sheets achieved the highest cumulative score with the combined factors. The final recommendation was that a safe workplace and a safe system of work are as important as equipment selection.

MDA (1997)

This study described a product evaluation of sixteen different handling products for moving dependent people in bed. The product types included:

1   sliding sheets;
2   short, low-friction rollers;
3   long, low-friction rollers; and
4   handling devices.

The products were allocated on a random basis and left with the carer and patient for a period of one week. The outcome data were collected using a questionnaire and interview.

The authors found that short, low-friction rollers were favoured over the other groups for moving people in bed. Named products were recommended for each group.

Owen and Hasler-Hanson (1999)

This study compared the perceived exertion felt by subjects when using three techniques to reposition a patient up the bed:

1   drawsheet;
2   slide-sheet one, single with handles; and
3   slide-sheet two, double sheet.

RPE was used as a measurement criterion as well as subjective patient data.

The results showed that the double slide-sheet required the least exertion and was the most secure. The drawsheet was found to be the most hazardous with significantly higher ratings for physical exertion. Slide-sheets were recommended for both patients and nurses.

Pain et al. (1999)

This quasi-experiment looked at fifteen non-mechanical devices to gain the views of carers about the functioning and ease of use. A questionnaire was used to get the carers' opinions, although the method of trialling the equipment was not clear.

The results showed that short, low-friction rollers had the highest overall rating. In general carers reported that products eased the task of moving dependent people in bed.

Robertson (2000)

This study aimed to produce guidelines for safe transfer slide-sheet use by measuring the amount of force required to move people of different weights up the bed or onto their sides using one or two slide-sheets. A spring balance was used to measure the force generated.

The results showed that two transfer sheets were needed when the full length of the patient was being moved up the bed. Two slide-sheets, or a folded slide-sheet, required less force to turn subjects of all weights. A slide-sheet under a bed sheet was less effective for heavy patients.

Tracy (1997)

This paper described a rough experiment to produce a purchasing recommendation for non-padded, roller slide-sheets. Data were collected using a spring balance to measure the horizontal force needed to initiate movement with a subject sitting on the slide-sheet.

Three named products were included in the recommendation.

Wright et al. (1991)

This study aimed to design and evaluate a new patient-lifting device – a lifting sheet with handles. The study took place both in a laboratory setting and 'on the job'. The main outcome measures were a questionnaire and measurement of EMG of the erector spinae and flexor digitorum muscles.

The results were conflicting about grip strength, and showed that the stress on the back was not significantly different. The device gave greater control and patient comfort.

Summary of evidence

Author and location	Subjects	Study type	QR	PR
Hignett (1999) UK	27 back-care advisors	quasi	57%	4.5
MDA (1997) UK	57 carers from acute, community and private homes	quasi	77%	4.0
Owen and Hasler-Hanson (1999) USA	5 nursing students	quasi	76%	5.0
Pain et al. (1999) UK	60 carers	quasi	50%	2.5

Robertson (2000) Australia	8 nurses	quasi	32%	3.0
Tracy (1997) UK	no detail	quasi	26%	3.0
Wright et al. (1991) USA	67 nursing students; 29 AICU/CICU nurses	quasi	35%	2.5

☺☺ Limited evidence that double (roller or two) slide-sheets are preferable to single sliding sheets

☺☺ Limited evidence that handles on slide-sheets do not alter the stress on the lower back

☺☺ Limited evidence that short, low-friction roller sheets are the preferred option for moving people in bed

7.2 HANDLING SLINGS

Section 7.2 summarises the evidence from three studies for handling slings, again from single studies so only offering limited-evidence level statements. A study from Australia found that using either one or two handling slings (with two carers) was preferable to a manual technique for chair–bed transfer and a paper from the UK reported that design criteria should include wider and padded handling slings. A handling sling is a length of flexible material with handles at either end, which lengthens the arm reach of the carer when positioned around or under a patient. It enhances the carer's technique by enabling them to bring the patient's centre of gravity closer. A sling may be used by one or two carers (MDA: A19, 1996).

Elford et al. (2000)

This quasi-experiment evaluated whether the use of patient-handling slings for lifting a patient from one seat to another reduced the risk of injury to the lumbar spine, compared with a similar technique without slings. Both one-sling and two-sling techniques were examined. Outcome measures were angular displacement and velocity measured with an LMM, and body-part stress rating.

Angular displacement showed lower values for both one and two slings than for no slings. Since the sling effectively lengthened the carer's arm length the amount of trunk flexion decreased. However the experiment only measured angles and not forces, so could not be applied to reducing the risk of injury. Subjectively the subjects preferred one or two slings to none.

Kothiyal and Yven (2000)

This study evaluated the muscle strain experienced by nursing staff during the transfer of a patient from a shower chair to a low chair with and without using a handling sling. Muscular strain was measured using EMG to erector spinae, although exactly how and where the electrodes were applied was not clear. Also RPE scale was used to gauge the subject's perception.

The use of a handling sling did not lead to any significant difference in muscle activity of erector spinae or trapezius (left or right) and there was a significant increase in perceived exertion on shoulder and lower back when the device was used. The authors recommended that patient-handling slings should be adjustable and attention should be given to the anthropometry of users.

MDA (1996)

This study identified which transferring equipment was best suited to the needs of carers and patients with various disabilities either in a private home or an institutional setting. They included:

1   three handling belts;
2   three handling slings;
3   two turntables; and
4   four sitting transfer boards.

The equipment was randomly allocated and left with the carer/patient partnership for a one-week period, and then evaluated using a questionnaire.

The results for Sections 1, 3 and 4 are reported in Sections 7.3 and 7.4. A preference was expressed for handling slings with greater width and made of a flexible material.

Summary of evidence

Author and location	Subjects	Study type	QR	PR
Elford et al. (2000) Australia	23 nurses	quasi	76%	3.5
Kothiyal and Yven (2000) Australia	10 nurses	quasi	32%	4.0
MDA (1996) UK	48 carer/patient partnerships	quasi	70%	4.0

☺☺   Limited evidence that using one or two handling slings with two carers is preferable to no slings

☺☺   Limited evidence that wider and padded handling slings are preferred

7.3   HANDLING/LIFTING/WALKING/GAIT BELTS

Nine studies are included in Section 7.3 with respect to handling belts. Descriptions of the different types of belt are included in as much detail as was given in the original paper. There are basically three different types of belts:

1   back belt: worn by carer to reduce personal risk;
2   lifting belt: worn by carer to assist patient to stand; and
3   handling/walking/gait belt: worn by patient to improve the handhold for the carer to assist with standing, walking, etc. It may be a band of flexible material with an adjustable fastening with vertical or horizontal handles (MDA: A19, 1996).

This section also includes a paper referring to lifting (back) belts, where the belt is worn by the carer rather than the patient where this was considered an option for the patient to pull up on when foot space was limited. There was moderate evidence from several studies to indicate that not only should two carers use handling belts but also that they should not be used by one carer alone. Evidence about the use of handling belts is conflicting with high-quality studies suggesting that walking belts are better than mechanical hoists but also others suggesting that the use of walking belts may result in higher compressive forces than other manual or mechanical techniques.

Benevolo et al. *(1993)*

This study looked at five methods of transferring a patient between a bed and a wheelchair:

1   classical manual method with one carer (stand in front, lock knees, grip patient by arms/armpits, lift and transfer);
2   classical manual method with two carers (stand at the side of the patient, grip under armpits and elbows, lift and transfer);
3   walking belt with one carer (hold handles on walking belt, block knees, rock, pull and transfer);
4   walking belt with two carers (stand in front/side, block foot, bend knees, grip belt and stabilise with other hand on wheelchair, rock, pull, lift and transfer); and
5   mechanical hoist.

The outcome measures included RPE; perceived safety (by carer and nurse); patient comfort; preferential ranking of transfer type by carer; and time for each transfer.

The authors found that the walking belt with two carers was the most efficient for all the measures, followed by the mechanical hoist and walking belt with one carer.

Gagnon et al. (1986)

This study looked at three methods of raising a patient from a chair with one carer:

1   with the hands;
2   with forearms behind the patient's back at shoulder level; and
3   with a belt held at waist level.

The forces acting on the lumbar spine at L5/S1 were estimated using EMG (erector spinae and oblique externals), video, force platform and measurement of the lever arm from photographs.

The authors found that the technique with the belt (3) was the most strenuous with respect to compressive forces, whereas the manual technique (1) had the lowest compression forces. The use of the belt was associated with higher levels of both internal and external work than the other two methods due to the different motion pattern characteristics at the beginning of the move and the longer lifting time.

Garg et al. (1991a and b), Garg and Owen (1994)

This laboratory study looked at the task of transferring a patient from a bed, shower chair and toilet to a wheelchair using eight different techniques (five manual methods were used):

1   lifting with two carers (drag);
2   rocking and pulling the patient with a gait belt (5 cm wide, no handles) and two carers;
3   rocking and pulling the patient with a sling (flexible polymer, 20.5 cm long, 50 cm wide with cut-outs for handles at each end) and one carer;
4   rocking and pulling the patient with a walking belt (12.5 cm, handles on each side) and one carer;
5   rocking and pulling the patient with a walking belt and two carers;
6–8   three different makes of mechanical hoists were used.

The outcome measures included: biomechanical evaluations (body angles, pulling forces), nine-point-rated perceived exertion scale, comfort and security ratings for patients; suitability of method for patients condition; carers' overall preference; transfer time.

The authors found that the use of a mechanical aid did not necessarily reduce the stress as two of the hoists took longer than some of the manual techniques. Their recommendation was to use the walking belt with two carers and a gentle rocking/pulling motion for weight-bearing patients and one of the hoists for non-weight-bearing, heavy or combative patients for a wheelchair to/from shower chair transfer.

Lavender et al. (1995)

This quasi-experiment hypothesised that trunk motions would be affected by the use of lifting belts (worn by the carer); that the combination of belt and stepping would lead to least trunk motion in transverse and frontal plane; and that variability in trunk motion would be reduced with the lifting belt. An LMM was used to measure trunk position, velocity and acceleration.

The findings were that lateral bending motions were reduced by the belt, but the effects were moderated by asymmetry and foot motions. The belt reduced lateral bending only when the feet did not move. The belt decreased peak lateral bending velocity and acceleration with increased asymmetry; there was an additional decrease with foot movement. The belt minimised transverse (twisting) motion regardless of foot motion. The recommendations were that lifting belts were beneficial in reducing lateral bending and twisting motions, but foot motion could eliminate most of the lateral bending and twisting. So lifting belts were useful where there was no space for foot motion.

MDA (1996)

This identified transferring equipment which was best suited to the needs of carers and patients with various disabilities either in a private home or an institutional setting. They included:

1   three handling belts;
2   three handling slings;
3   two turntables; and
4   four sitting transfer boards.

The equipment was randomly allocated and left with the carer/patient partnership for a one-week period, and then evaluated using a questionnaire.

The results for Sections 2, 3 and 4 are reported in Sections 7.2 and 7.4. The belts were generally found to be useful if the patient was difficult to hold securely, had difficulty bending at the hip, or had poor trunk control. A preference was expressed for diagonally secured belts (female patients); wider, padded belts; with a 'velcro' fastening rather than a buckle; and with a horizontal handle.

Pan and Freivalos (2000)

This quasi-experiment evaluated a turntable with a frame in biomechanical terms and compared it to existing handling devices (a walking belt and a mechanical lift). The outcome measures used were EMG, heart rate, RPE, biomechanical analysis (video – compressive forces) and time taken.

The results showed that the walking belt exceeded the NIOSH recommended limits. The framed turntable was better overall than the belt but not as good as the powered lifter.

Ulin et al. (1997)

This study looked at transfers from bed to wheelchair for two totally dependent patients (light and heavy) using six methods, all performed with two carers:

1   pivot transfer;
2   gait belt;
3   sliding board;
4   screw-actuated lift;
5   hydraulic lift; and
6   electric lift.

The outcome measures included RPE; compressive force on L5/S1 using a 3D static strength prediction programme; force gauge to determine the force required to roll or position the patient and pump the hoist; hand force; and posture modelling.

The authors found that low-back compressive forces exceeded the back compression NIOSH limits for manual methods but not for mechanical methods. No difference was found in RPE between light and heavy patients for manual methods. The authors predicted that less than 4 per cent of the female population would have the strength at the hip to perform the transfer using the gait belt, and for all the manual methods less than 53 per cent of the female population would have sufficient strength to carry out the transfer.

The authors recommended that a mechanical lift should be used to transfer totally dependent patients from a bed to a wheelchair regardless of patient weight.

Summary of evidence

Author and location	Subjects	Study type	QR	PR
Benevolo et al. (1993) Italy	6 nurses and 6 physiotherapists	quasi	57%	4.0
Gagnon et al. (1986) Canada	6 male nursing students	quasi	57%	4.0
Garg et al. (1991a) USA	6 nursing students	quasi	80%	4.5

Garg et al. (1991b) USA	6 nursing students	quasi	48%	4.0
Garg and Owen (1994) USA	57 nursing assistants	quasi	67%	4.5
Lavender et al. (1995) USA	16 nurses and nursing students	quasi	63%	4.0
MDA (1996) UK	48 carer/patient partnerships	quasi	70%	4.0
Pan and Freivalos (2000) USA	6 subjects (no detail)	quasi	33%	3.0
Ulin et al. (1997) USA	2 nurses	quasi	67%	5.0

☺☺☺   Moderate evidence from two studies for using a walking belt with two carers for weight-bearing patients

☺☺☺   Moderate evidence from two studies for not using a walking belt with one carer for weight-bearing patients

☺☺   Limited evidence that wider, padded belts with 'velcro' fastening and a horizontal handle are preferred

☺☺   Limited evidence that lifting belts (worn by the carer) may be useful if there if no space for foot motion

7.4   SLIDING (TRANSFER) BOARDS AND TURNTABLES

This section considers sliding-boards and turntables. A sliding-board is a piece of flat rigid material which is placed between two surfaces to allow a patient to slide between the two (MDA: A19, 1996). A turntable consists of two circular discs which are fixed centrally and rotate on each other. It is placed under the feet (generally hard turntable) or under the bottom (generally soft turntable) of the patient (MDA: A19, 1996).

Two limited-evidence statements are given with respect to the thickness of turntables and the shape of sitting sliding-boards.

MDA (1996)

This study identified which transferring equipment was best suited to the needs of carers and patients with various disabilities either in a private home or an institutional setting. They included:

1   three handling belts;
2   three handling slings;
3   two turntables; and
4   four sitting sliding-boards.

The equipment was randomly allocated and left with the carer/patient partnership for a one-week period, and then evaluated using a questionnaire.

The results for Sections 1 and 2 are reported in Sections 7.2 and 7.3. The thinner turntables were preferred with a diameter sufficiently large to fit the patients' feet. Longer and wider sitting transfer-boards were found to be more stable, but were also difficult to position. Straight boards were preferred to curved boards for both use and storage.

Pan and Freivalos (2000)

This quasi-experiment evaluated a sit–stand–turn device (Williamson Medical Devices, Ford City, PA) in biomechanical terms and compared it to existing handling devices, a walking belt and a mechanical lift. The outcome measures used were EMG, heart rate, RPE, biomechanical analysis (video – compressive forces) and time taken.

The results showed that the walking belt exceeded the NIOSH recommended limits. The sit–stand–turn was better overall than the belt but not as good as the powered lifter.

Zelenka et al. (1996)

An analysis of the efficiency, with respect to the force required, of commercially available transfer devices suitable for the task of a lateral horizontal transfer between a bed and trolley (gurney) was undertaken. The three devices were:

1   a patient roller: a frame of five rollers with a plastic cover which is rolled under the patient as they are pulled between the surfaces;
2   a patient shifter: a thin, semi-rigid plastic board with four handles cut along each side. The patient is moved with patient shifter between surfaces, so it is not a bridging board; and
3   a drawsheet.

Four hundred and fifty transfers were carried out with the three devices. Force scales were used to measure the maximum forces required.

The study found that the patient roller required a consistently lower force (44 per cent less) than the shifter or drawsheet regardless of the direction of force applied. The patient shifter, in turn, required less force than the drawsheet. The patient roller was recommended.

Summary of evidence

Author and location	Subjects	Study type	QR	PR
MDA (1996) UK	48 carer/patient partnerships	quasi	70%	4.0
Pan and Freivalos (2000) USA	6 subjects (no detail)	quasi	33%	3.0
Zelenka et al. (1996) USA	15 hospital workers and office staff	quasi	48%	3.5

☺☺ Limited evidence that thinner turntables are preferred

☺☺ Limited evidence that straight, sitting–sliding transfer boards are preferred to curved boards

7.5 ATTITUDES TOWARDS/PERCEPTIONS OF SMALL AIDS

Four studies are included which look at attitudes and perceptions about small aids. The findings indicate that the equipment availability influences use and tends to back up evidence seen elsewhere that many factors influence risk reduction rather than just equipment provision.

Bewick and Gardner (2000)

This survey investigated a range of factors in the safety of nursing aides, including knowledge of safe manual handling, attitudes and beliefs and the use of mechanical aids. A questionnaire was used.

The results showed that the respondents had a good knowledge of safe manual handling and used aids 50 per cent of the time.

The reasons given for not using aids were that the patient was light, they were sure of their own ability and that no mechanical aids were available. The study recommended that equipment should be fitted to the task and suggested that training and equipment alone would not solve the problem.

Owen (1988)

This survey set out to identify which patient-handling devices were in use and how frequently they were used for which tasks. The devices mentioned in the paper were:

1   hydraulic lift;
2   gait belt;
3   lift sheet;
4   bed trapeze (lifting pole);
5   patient roller;
6   sliding-board;
7   turntable;
8   rope ladder; and
9   bathtub lift.

The author used a questionnaire to collect the data.

The results found that the gait belt was the most frequently used (64 per cent), followed by the bathtub lift (59 per cent), lift sheet (52 per cent), hydraulic lift (34 per cent) and that the rope ladder and turntable were rarely used. The task for which devices were most commonly used was bed–chair transfers followed by to/from the bathtub and lifting up the bed. The common problems experienced included the time involved to use a device, staff experience and lack of availability of devices.

Panciera et al. (2000)

This professional opinion looked at patient-lifting devices, hygiene aids and minor aids. It gave a logical and well-referenced account to set out a procedure for choosing aids and suggested that an adequate supply of all aids, appropriately adapted to each situation, was one of the most effective means of reducing risk.

Scott (1995)

This qualitative study set out to discover what factors in the working environment created difficulties for nursing staff, and to investigate nurses' own perceptions of their problems and ability to cope when moving patients. A questionnaire with both open and closed questions was used.

The findings raised issues around staffing levels, lack of space, time and knowledge.

Summary of evidence

Author and location	Subjects	Study type	QR	PR
Bewick and Gardner (2000) Australia	50 nursing aides	x-sect.	55%	4.0
Owen (1988) USA	175 licensed long-care facilities	survey	57%	4.0
Panciera et al. (2000) Italy	—	PO	PO	3.5
Scott (1995) UK	85 nurses	qual.	8%	1.0

☺☺   Limited evidence that the availability of equipment will influence its use in practice

☺☺   Limited evidence that the gait belt is the most commonly used small handling aid

CHAPTER 8

BEDS

This chapter reviews the literature available about beds and cots in a variety of environments.

8.1 BED HEIGHT

Seven studies are included in this section. There is moderate evidence from two good-quality studies and three lower-quality studies to support the use of adjustable-height beds, although the height should be set for individual preference with respect to the task being undertaken.

Baglioni (1999)

This professional opinion detailed the response to a presidential decree requesting accreditation of health facilities in Italy. It described an analysis of working tasks relative to patients which highlighted improvements or detrimental effects of environmental characteristics.

The author recommended that beds should have:

1   bigger handles to help patients to move;
2   height adjustment from 40 to 70 cm;
3   brakes;
4   supporting legs designed such that they do not impede wheelchairs;
5   supports for the head and foot boards; and
6   adjustments and tilt in three sections.

Botha and Bridger (1998)

This survey looked at whether pain and usability problems with beds were related to the body dimensions of nurses. Observation techniques as well as measurement of the workplace and anthropometric measurements were used.

The survey found that the height of the bed was dependent on the task and that 34 per cent of subjects found the range of height-adjustable beds sufficient. Thirty-four per cent found it difficult to adjust the height, and 49 per cent found the beds too heavy to move around. Trapped fingers in cot-sides (68 per cent) or when adjusting the bed (59 per cent) were reported.

Caboor et al. (2000)

This controlled trial investigated the implications on spinal motion, muscular activity and perceived exertion when nurses were given the opportunity to choose bed heights during typical nursing tasks. Four standardised tasks were investigated with a standard-height bed and with an individually-adjusted bed:

1   turning a patient and inserting a bed pan;
2   washing;
3   transferring to and from a seated position; and
4   transferring in and out of bed.

A spinal motion monitor, EMG and RPE were used as measures.

The results showed no significant changes in the measurement criteria suggesting that the range of motion was not influenced by the bed height. However the results may have been limited as the standardised bed height was close to optimal for most subjects and the average bed-height adjustment was only 0.064 m.

De Looze et al. (1994)

This quasi-experiment determined the effects of individually chosen bed-height adjustments on various estimates of mechanical low-back stress. The following tasks were performed at a fixed height of 0.715 m and at a variable height adjusted by subjects:

1   turning a lying patient;
2   repositioning the patient up the bed;
3   helping a patient sitting on the edge of the bed to standing and vice versa.

A biomechanical model was used to calculate joint movement and joint reaction forces (compression and shear).

Significant favourable effects of bed height adjustment were observed for the time-integrated compression and shear and for peak shear force. Lower peak values for compression force with bed-height adjustment were observed, but were insignificant. This showed a reduction in exposure to a high level of force on L5/S1 motion segments without a rise in peak force. Therefore the use of height-adjustable beds was supported, and their effect on subsequent low-back problems depended on the nurses' capacity to adjust the height of the bed.

De Looze et al. (1998)

The paper investigated the question of whether strength affected performance for three tasks carried out at two bed heights. The following tasks were performed at a fixed height of 0.715 m and at a variable height adjusted by subjects:

1   turning a lying patient;
2   pulling/lifting a patient from sitting on the edge of the bed into standing;
3   lowering the patient from standing to sitting on the edge of the bed.

Elbow, knee and trunk strength were measured using a 2D segmental model which included ground reaction forces (using a force plate), kinematic data (markers on the joints), and anthropometric data.

The authors found that the task performance was not affected by the strength of the individual nurse and that the adjustment of the bed height by the nurses did not correlate with their individual body height.

Lee and Chiou (1994)

This study looked at psychophysically determined MAPH (maximum acceptable capacity in patient-handling tasks) in kilograms at three bed heights (70 cm, 80 cm and iliac crest height) for five tasks:

1   horizontal lifting of a dummy to the bed side;
2   turning the dummy from supine to side-lying;
3   turning from side-lying to prone;
4   turning from prone to side-lying; and
5   turning from side-lying to supine.

The outcome measures included RPE and MAPH.

The authors found no significant difference between the MAPH at 80 cm and iliac crest height. The highest exertion was perceived with the 70-cm bed height. They concluded that matching the job demands (bed height) to a person's characteristics was effective in reducing the risks in patient handling.

Nestor (1988)

This pilot cross-sectional survey determined the effect of existing hospital-bed design on the incidence rates of low-back pain among nursing personnel in a hospital setting. Bed-height cycle times and nursing-control location were recorded and compared with the incidence of low-back pain.

The results indicated that long bed-cycle times and controls at the foot of the bed might explain increased incidence of LBP. The most useful hospital bed had a cycle time of approximately 20 seconds, with the controls on the bed side-frame or side-rail.

Summary of evidence

Author and location	Subjects	Study type	QR	PR
Baglioni (1999) Italy	none described	PO	PO	4.0
Botha and Bridger (1998) South Africa	100 nurses	survey	75%	5.0
Caboor et al. (2000) Belgium/Netherlands	18 nurses	quasi	61%	3.5
De Looze et al. (1994) Netherlands	22 nurses	quasi	72%	5.0
De Looze et al. (1998) Netherlands	17 nurses	quasi	66%	4.0
Lee and Chiou (1994) Taiwan	24 female nurses	quasi	39%	3.5
Nestor (1988) USA	1133 nurses from 3 hospitals	x-sect.	50%	2.5

☺☺☺   Moderate evidence from three studies to support the use of adjustable-height beds for caring tasks

☺☺   Limited evidence from one study that the location of the bed controls and bed-height cycle time may be associated with the incidence of low-back pain

8.2   ELECTRIC BEDS AND COTS

The use of electric beds was explored in four studies. The evidence is graded as limited due to the lack of high-quality studies. However there is evidence that electric beds promote patient independence for in-bed tasks, movement and access/egress.

Dhoot and Georgieva (1996)

This study aimed to determine the potential for electric beds to reduce manual handling and increase the quality of care in comparison with hydraulic variable-height (Kings Fund) beds. Observational data were collected about the frequency with which:

1   the patient used the functions of the bed; and
2   the nurses were involved in the use of the bed functions.

The authors found that the electric bed increased patient independence and considerably reduced the physical strain that the nurses were subjected to when lifting patients manually.

Hampton (1998)

This controlled experiment considered pressure care and quality of care, suggesting that the use of electric features of the bed would encourage patient independence in getting in and out of bed as well as decrease the number of nurses involved in handling the patient. The intervention group was supplied with electrically-operated beds with pressure mattresses for six months. A structured questionnaire measured the nurses' and patients' evaluation of patient comfort, ease of mobility and ease of manual handling.

Sixty-five per cent of nurses in the experimental group found it easier to transfer the patients and 63 per cent achieved 'no lifting'. The study recommended the use of electric beds to achieve a no-lifting policy.

Kitson (2000)

This professional opinion detailed the development and use of electric variable-height paediatric cots. It was suggested that this equipment resulted in a marked reduction in the need to bend over the cot.

Mitchell et al. (1998)

This booklet reported on the Kings Fund centenary bed project to review the design specification for the 'Kings Fund' bed. Wide consultation was reported with representatives from NHS hospital Trusts (acute and community), private health-care providers, self-help disability support and professional organisations, as well as manufacturers.

Guidelines were produced for the design and selection of beds for hospitals, nursing and residential-care and private homes. All areas were recommended to consider using powered profiling (at least powered back rest), variable-height beds for patients with limited or compromised mobility.

Summary of evidence

Author and location	Subjects	Study type	QR	PR
Dhoot and Georgieva (1996) UK	4 nurses	quasi	59%	4.0
Hampton (1998) UK	782 patients on 2 wards	quasi	76%	3.5
Kitson (2000) UK	—	PO	PO	4.0
Mitchell et al. (1998) UK	no detail	PO	PO	4.0

☺☺☺ Moderate evidence from two studies that electric beds reduce the physical strain relating to nursing manual-handling tasks associated with caring for patients in bed

☺☺ Limited evidence to support the use of electric beds for patients to increase independence and in-bed mobility

CHAPTER 9

HOISTS

This chapter summarises the literature which was found with respect to using hoists and the design of hoists and slings. Studies where hoists were part of, or the main factor of, an intervention have been reported in Chapter 11.

9.1 USING HOISTS

Nine studies are included in this section, with four having a QR of ≥50 per cent. They investigated why hoists are not used to their full capacity. A number of complex reasons were identified which included staff attitudes, management attitude, lack of knowledge (and training) about the equipment and difficulties in applying slings. Some of these issues are addressed in Sections 9.2 and 9.3 which review the studies on hoist and sling designs.

Bell (1987)

This narrative review (professional opinion) described how mechanical hoists for lifting patients have been available for one hundred years but suggested that they are not being used. The author put forward the following reasons for non-use:

1 time;
2 effort/trouble;
3 patients' dislike of the equipment;
4 devices not readily available;
5 low level of knowledge about the devices;
6 restricted space to use the hoists;
7 equipment (e.g. beds, chairs) not compatible with hoists; and
8 low motivation to use the devices.

The author recommended that attention to the patient/carer/task/environment interfaces was essential to both the equipment design and selection.

McGuire and Dewar (1995)

This survey looked at:

1   the extent of training; and
2   the use of mechanical aids, using a postal questionnaire to collect data.

The authors found that 60.5 per cent of the study population did not use mechanical aids in all the appropriate situations they encountered, because 24 per cent felt they were unsuitable, 14 per cent did not have them available and 10 per cent reported inconvenient locations. Only 35 per cent considered themselves able to move and handle the equipment correctly but only for about 50 per cent of their working time.

McGuire et al. (1996a)

This paper described a survey which was carried out to identify patients' views about the mechanical aids used to move them and how they compared to nurses' perceived views. Data were collected using semi-structured interviews with patients and ward observations of mechanical aid activity.

The authors found that despite the fact that most patients did not object to the use of mechanical aids (90 per cent), staff still stated that they did not use them because patients didn't like them (in fact only 10 per cent); other reasons given were that they take too long and that they were unsuitable for certain situations. The authors suggested that the problem of use of mechanical aids rests with nurses' attitudes.

McGuire et al. (1997)

This study was carried out to identify the attitudes of management and finance staff to the health and safety of hospital nursing staff when considering the use of mechanical aids in the ward. A questionnaire was used to collect data.

The authors found that the allocation of funds was a lower priority with respect to decreasing back injuries and that training and equipment took higher priority. They suggested that clearer guidelines were required about funding/ purchase of hoists as different levels/types of staff showed a lack of knowledge about their own or others' responsibility in the provision, use and maintenance of hoists. They also suggested that there was an inappropriate emphasis on training.

Meyer (1995)

This study investigated the lack of use of hoists using a questionnaire.

The findings reported include: 41 per cent found hoists too large, bulky, unwieldy or had insufficient space in which to use them; 32 per cent had no access to maintenance; 62 per cent had no access to instructions.

Moody et al. (1996)

This exploratory interview study looked at nurses' attitudes towards mechanical aids (mobile hoists, fixed hoists, standard hoists, bath hoists and overhead hoists). Data were collected using interviews.

The authors found that the perceived safety and comfort of the mechanical aids were related to the favourability with which the nurses viewed the mechanical aid. There were a number of factors identified which might change the use of the hoist: training (83 per cent had no formal training); 57 per cent did not know the maximum weight limit of the hoist; 59 per cent did not know who was responsible for laundering slings; 57 per cent found difficulties in attaching the slings. Only 59 per cent felt the use of a mechanical aid resulted in less exertion although 87 per cent thought they were safer for nursing staff. They concluded by saying that mechanical aids were not used to a significant extent due to complex reasons, but that equipment-specific training and addressing ward-specific practical problems would help to increase usage.

Newman and Callaghan (1993)

This survey by postal questionnaire investigated the availability of mechanical handling aids, the frequency of their use and reasons for non-use.

The authors found that 65.5 per cent of those surveyed said that they had lifting aids available and 83 per cent used the aids.

Switzer and Porter (1993)

This qualitative study observed the lifting behaviour of nurses in wards where hoists were available to find out how nurses felt about using hoists.

The results showed a continued use of unsafe lifts due to factors such as the lack of training in hoist use and passing on bad practice. They also reported the nurses' feelings that they were not consulted about the choice of hoists or smaller equipment. There was a perceived conflict in providing comfort and dignity and the need to use equipment to improve safety.

Takala and Kukkonen (1987)

This survey looked at the use of lifting aids and the role of lifting instructions and training on a ward. Seven wards in five hospitals were surveyed. The outcome measures included questionnaires, interviews and video analysis. The results showed that mechanical hoists were only used where the ward had well organised, on-the-job training and management support. Video analysis of hoist use showed that they were slower that manual alternatives by 3–6 per cent of an eight-hour shift (15–29 minutes).

Summary of evidence

Author and location	Subjects	Study type	QR	PR
Bell (1987) UK	—	PO	PO	3.5
McGuire and Dewar (1995) UK	3548 nurses	survey	39%	4.0
McGuire et al. (1996a) UK	23 patients	survey	50%	3.5
McGuire et al. (1997) UK	43 NHS hospital trusts	survey	64%	5.0
Meyer (1995) Germany	7 care institutions and hospitals	survey	32%	4.0
Moody et al. (1996) UK	185 nurses	survey	41%	4.0
Newman and Callaghan (1993) UK	173 nurses and midwives	survey	39%	4.0
Switzer and Porter (1993) New Zealand	37 nurses	qual.	62%	4.5
Takala and Kukkonen (1987) Finland	143 nurses	survey	50%	3.5

☺☺☺ Moderate evidence from four studies that there are complex reasons why hoists are not used to their full capacity. These reasons include staff attitude, lack of training, lack of availability, lack of knowledge about hoists, difficulties in attaching slings, and lack of space

9.2 HOIST DESIGN

Seven studies are included in this section. Three have a QR of ≥50 per cent. One indicates a need for training, a second makes a product-purchasing recommendation and the third looks at overhead hoists. As all three address different research questions the evidence statements are at the limited level.

Bell (1984)

This survey described the types of problems encountered by nursing staff when using hoists and sought identifying criteria to improve hoist selection and utilisation. Outcome measures and smaller studies designed to answer the questions included the manoeuvrability of hoists, training and changes in performance, and time taken to use the hoist.

The findings showed that hoist manoeuvrability could be much improved by careful alignment of castors during assembly. Participants who attended teaching sessions were faster and more accurate in using the hoists. The study recommended the appointment of a nursing-equipment officer, teaching packages for hoists and other lifting aids, and on-going research into the development and manufacture of lifting aids.

Hignett (1998)

This quasi-experiment/user trial aimed to give a purchasing recommendation for electric, mobile hoists to promote the standardisation of hoisting equipment throughout a large, acute teaching hospital. Twelve different hoists were each used in eight trials. The outcome measures included individual rating and group ranking of product features, time taken and RPE.

The findings resulted in a named manufacturer/product as the purchasing recommendation.

LeBon and Forrester (1996)

This quasi-experiment evaluated the 'elevate and transfer vehicle' when used to transfer an adult from one seated position to another. The outcome measures included expert appraisal, user trials and performance tests.

The results found that the device needed some design improvements with patients finding it undignified and unstable.

Love (1996b)

This professional opinion offered a description of how to use and select hoists. The author stated that hoists must be stable and strong, and used for transfers, not for transport. There must not be a mismatch with the physical environment.

McGuire et al. (1996b)

This experiment evaluated the acceptability and effectiveness of a range of mechanical aids in a laboratory setting using trained nurses and carers as subjects. The outcome measures were performance criteria including use of brakes, spreader bars, safety and stability, speed of lowering and raising, etc.

The main findings were that attention needed to be given to design issues, and to training.

Olsson and Brandt (1992)

This survey looked at the use of ceiling-mounted hoists by eighteen users in private homes from nine different manufacturers. The main outcome measure was a questionnaire.

The results showed that there was a need for improvements in the design of hoists especially regarding the spreader bar and sling attachment. There was also a need for improvement in the instructions given to carers especially with respect to the selection of type and size of sling.

Quintana and Alonso (1997)

This professional opinion described the development of an overhead hoisting system attached to a bed. The gantry used a monorail with two trolleys (spreader bars) for hammock lifting. The prototype was evaluated for back safety (NIOSH), nurse productivity (time saved) and cost analysis (return on investment).

The authors reported that the back safety was much improved, the productivity saved an estimated 96 minutes per shift and an estimated 20.1 per cent return on investment would be found (to include sickness absence, cost of development, etc.).

Summary of evidence

Author and location	Subjects	Study type	QR	PR
Bell (1984) UK	26 students (no details)	quasi	33%	4.0
Hignett (1998) UK	16 nurses and occupational therapists	survey	59%	5.0
LeBon and Forrester (1996) Australia	11 hospital staff	quasi	41%	3.0

Love (1996b) UK	—	PO	PO	2.5
McGuire et al. (1996b) UK	nurses (n = ?)	quasi	54%	3.0
Olsson and Brandt (1992) Denmark	218,611 patient homes	survey	75%	3.0
Quintana and Alonso (1997) USA	no detail	PO	PO	3.0

☺☺☺ Moderate evidence that hoist design (mobile and overhead) can be improved

9.3   SLING DESIGN AND USE

Three studies looked at two different aspects of slings. For sling design there was moderate evidence from two good-quality studies which found that sling use and comfort were compromised by difficulties in:

1   selecting the correct size;
2   design of leg pieces; and
3   method of application.

The third study looked at the spreader bar design.

Edlund et al. *(1998)*

This study aimed to analyse how the hoist spreader-bar design affected the sitting position. They looked at twelve designs of spreader bars for three selected slings. Photographic data were collected and used to analyse the length of the supporting area, the shortest sagittal length, angle of inclination of the trunk, and the angle between the thighs and horizontal plane.

The authors found that all the spreader bars affected sitting angles and were affected by the sling design. The shorter-width spreader bar decreased the risk of falling forwards and offered a greater supporting area, whereas the longer spreader bars gave relatively upright sitting positions.

MDA (1994)

This MDA report described an evaluation of sixteen hoist slings. A range of different slings was used for the following transfers:

1   bed–chair;
2   chair–toilet;
3   bed–toilet;
4   chair–bath; and
5   bed–bath.

Data were collected using a questionnaire which asked about comfort, ease of use, design and effectiveness of the sling.

The authors found that 60 per cent of patients experienced some discomfort when being transferred, with the most common area being the back of the knee. Eighty-nine per cent of carers experienced some difficulties in using slings in their normal clinical practice. The listed difficulties included: time taken to put on/remove the sling; positioning the sling correctly; finding an effective sling to transfer a patient onto the toilet; preventing the material from digging into the patient.

Norton (2000)

This cross-sectional study reported an analysis of the form and structure of hoist slings as an interface in relation to their use by nurses and experience by patients. Data were collected by direct observation, interviews with staff and patients and an evaluation of the slings.

The author found that the patients' opinion with respect to the comfort of the sling appeared to be related to the use of the correct size and the method of application.

Summary of evidence

Author and location	Subjects	Study type	QR	PR
Edlund et al. (1998)	12 subjects (none nursing)	x-sect.	57%	4.5
MDA (1994) UK	18 carers	quasi	59%	4.0
Norton (2000) UK	9 nurses	x-sect.	67%	5.0

☺☺☺   Moderate evidence from two studies that sling use and comfort are compromised by difficulties in:

1   selecting the correct size;
2   design of leg pieces; and
3   method of application

☺☺   Limited evidence that spreader-bar design will affect the resultant sitting angle

SECTION IV

INTERVENTIONS

CHAPTER 10

TRAINING INTERVENTIONS

This chapter summarises the evidence available to support the use of training as the main factor of an intervention programme. Different outcome measures were used in the various studies; these have been grouped as those showing:

1   no benefit from training;
2   mixed results;
3   benefit from training.

The overall conclusion is that interventions which are predominantly based on training or education have no impact on working practices or injury rates.

10.1 STUDIES DESCRIBING TRAINING INTERVENTIONS WITH NO IMPACT ON WORKING PRACTICES OR INJURY RATES

Twenty studies from six countries are included in the first section. These were carried out between 1983 and 2001, and used a variety of methodologies including case series, quasi-experimental, cohort study, experiments, surveys, cross-sectional studies and professional opinions (as narrative literature reviews). The outcome measures included the risk and rate of injury; transfer of classroom skills to the work place; working postures; and physical fitness. All concluded, to a greater or lesser extent, that training (or education alone) had no effect on the outcome measures.

Billin (1998)

This study described an intervention for moving and handling in neuro-disability nursing using equipment and training. The author evaluated the interventions using retrospective analysis of moving and handling injury incidents.

The study found that the number of injury incidents increased over a five-year period (1992–7) but it was suggested that this was due to increased reporting rather than increased incidence (no evidence was presented for this conclusion). It was suggested that equipment and training had no effect on the number of moving and handling incidents.

Dietz and Baumann (2000)

This paper described an evaluation of a three-day training programme for nurses and physiotherapists over a three-year period. The course included two days on specific body movements and one day on practical applications. The impact was measured using a questionnaire. The authors found that 76 per cent felt that they had not learnt the basic positions at the end of the course and that 49 per cent felt the positions could not be used in their clinical work.

Engkvist et al. (2001)

This postal questionnaire investigated the interaction between single risk factors for back injuries and analysed how individual characteristics contributed to the risk of injuries in these situations.

The results were given for three risk indicators:

1   patient transfers: the risk neither increased with an increased number of transfers nor decreased with experience;
2   use of transfer devices: infrequent use of devices was associated with increased risk for full-time workers but not part-time workers; and
3   training: this was not associated with a decreased risk of injury.

Fanello et al. (1999)

This study described the evaluation of an education-based prevention programme on musculoskeletal disorders and working conditions and activities of health-care providers. The training programme lasted six days, and included principles of low-back-pain prevention and theoretical instruction. Refresher training was given at three and six months with two days of observation and feedback. The impact was measured in an intervention group and a control group with a questionnaire at the start (baseline) and after two years.

No difference was found between the two groups in the injury rate, amount of patient handling and static postures or musculoskeletal complaints. It was concluded that there was no impact from education alone.

Griffith and McArthur (1999)

This qualitative study looked at the perception of moving and handling training for care assistants. The training programme offered a seven-day course on induction (five days on general health and safety issues and two days on moving and handling), followed by a refresher of two half-days of theory and practice, four weeks apart. The training was evaluated using a questionnaire (including the GHQ), with the responses audio-taped.

The authors found that the care assistants had learnt about postural awareness and equipment but had not acquired transferable skills with respect to applying the techniques in different environments.

Harber et al. (1994)

This prospective study of newly trained nurses looked at which worksite and personal factors were likely to be predictors of future back pain. Data were collected using telephone interviews and written questionnaires.

They found that there was no association between training and back-pain prevention.

Hignett (1996b)

This narrative literature review summarises previous studies. The author suggested that there was little evidence to support technique training.

Johnston (1987)

This cross-sectional study investigated the hypothesis that student nurses would be safer if they were given extra instruction and supervision in the clinical area on how to assess patient mobility. The intervention was evaluated using a questionnaire to ask about the students' feelings with respect to the information and support they had received.

The results showed that there was a lack of instruction and supervision, with only 27.5 per cent of lifts being assessed and planned. The paper concluded by saying that there was little evidence of supervision of student nurses when moving and handling patients.

Lagerström and Hagberg (1997)

This three-year longitudinal study evaluated an education and training programme which included:

1   patient transfer techniques;
2   physical fitness exercises; and

3   stress management.

Data were collected with:

- questionnaires on posture;
- patient-transfer skill;
- physical fitness; and
- an RPE scale.

The results indicated that the techniques (and equipment use) taught on the programme were being used but that not only was there no reduction in the overall musculoskeletal injury prevalence but that hip and upper-back problems were increasing.

Nussbaum and Torres (2001)

Two different training approaches were examined to determine whether training leads to short-term decreases of known injury risk factors through quantifiable changes in behaviour. Training was provided using:

1   a twenty-five-minute training video; and
2   a two-hour lecture and practical session.

Outcome measures were RPE, posture, load location (horizontal distance of load from body) and biomechanical measures using a static model.

The authors found that overall training (both groups) had an effect (but not significant) on lifting postures. The video had the same effect as the lecture/practical session: there was no significant difference between groups, though a larger effect was seen with the lecture/practice group.

Raistrick (1981)

This survey compared the level of back injuries over twelve months before and after the implementation of a training programme. The programme included a range of techniques, e.g. orthodox lift, shoulder lift, through-arm lift and three-man lift.

No change was reported in the percentage of back injuries.

Rodgers (1985b)

The author described an exploration of the characteristics of a positive lifting and handling ward environment using a questionnaire survey and interviews to collect data.

The results showed that the nurses did not use the lifts taught in the school of nursing but that a ward method of lifting was in evidence. It was suggested that the simple, most important factor was the staff relationships which resulted in whether the ward was seen as 'positive' for lifting.

Scopa (1993)

This study used a comparison of two different methods of instruction:

1   classroom training; and
2   independent study in body mechanics.

The methods were evaluated by looking at the use of the techniques and any modifications in work-related body mechanics pre- and post-intervention.

No significant difference was found between the pre- and post-measures.

Stubbs et al. (1983)

This two-stage study looked at whether techniques could be successfully taught. The techniques (shoulder lift, orthodox lift, through-arm lift, and under-arm drag) were taught to two student nurses at four training sessions to give one-to-one instruction, group instruction, practice and testing sessions. The techniques were evaluated using IAP.

Results showed that there was minimal reduction in IAP at best, and deterioration at worst. The follow up, at fifteen weeks, showed poor retention of skills.

St Vincent et al. (1989)

This field study compared the taught handling methods for hospital orderlies with those subsequently used in the workplace. The aim was to determine whether the taught methods were used, with the main deviations characterised. Observational data were collected with a piloted observational grid.

The study concluded that training in the classroom rarely transferred to the work place and that training programmes were poorly adapted to handling operations carried out in a hospital environment.

Venning (1988)

This literature review sought to determine if education was an effective intervention in the primary prevention of work-related injuries. The literature review identified three major predictors of high risk as:

1   job factors (e.g. area of work);
2   job activities; and

3   job categories of practical nurses, aides and attendants.

The author concluded by saying that education alone would not solve the problem.

Troup and Rauhala (1987) and Videman et al. (1989)

These papers described the assessment of skills acquired by student nurses from a self-help education programme based on twenty hours of theory and practical teaching on moving and handling over four semesters (five hours per semester) using the first edition of *The Guide to the Handling of Patients* (Troup *et al.*, 1981). The students were encouraged to evaluate their learned skills using self-evaluation videos and diaries of patient-handling activities. Two groups had the new training and two groups continued with the old-style training (content not described). The acquisition of skills was assessed on a bed–commode transfer, where the students had a choice of handling aids (including hoist, small aids) and could ask for assistance.

The results showed that 93 per cent of the intervention group had acquired new skills in comparison with 65 per cent of the control group. Lifting aids were used by 53 per cent of the intervention group compared with 2 per cent of the control group. But both groups rated relatively low for patient-handling skills. There was no statistical difference between the groups for back injuries.

Wachs and Parker (1987)

This observation study investigated how nurses moved patients in bed to establish whether prescribed techniques were being used. A thirteen-point checklist/observation guide to identify environmental and carer factors was used.

The study found that the nurses did not move the patients in bed as they had been taught. For example the bed height was not adjusted; side rails were not lowered; they did not rock to aid movement; they did not flex their knees to keep their backs straight. Only 17 per cent of the observed postures were prescribed (low prevalence of lifting behaviour), whereas 23 per cent of the postures were labelled as being at risk of low-back pain.

Wood (1987)

This study was an evaluation of a back programme in a geriatric hospital which aimed to lower the incidence of back injuries through a feedback-oriented educational programme. Feedback was given on correct techniques rather than formal classes on new material by:

1   assessing individual lifting ability for one- and two-carer transfers;
2   observation of the tasks of bed bathing, bed–wheelchair transfer, dressing and putting patient to bed; and

3   one-hour classroom demonstration of body mechanics, lift and transfer techniques and proper use of equipment.

No significant difference was found between the control and experimental groups, suggesting that that the back programme was not effective, although the staff perceived it to be good.

Summary of evidence

Author and location	Subjects	Study type	QR	PR
Billin (1998) UK	nurses, occupational therapists and physiotherapists (n = ?)	quasi	54%	2.0
Dietz and Baumann (2000) France	103 nurses and physiotherapists	quasi	33%	3.5
Engkvist et al. (2001) Sweden	292 nurses	case	100%	5.0
Fanello et al. (1999) France	272 non-clerical hospital staff	quasi	80%	5.0
Griffith and McArthur (1999) UK	502 health care assistants	qual.	42%	3.0
Harber et al. (1994) USA	179 newly qualified nurses	cohort	73%	4.5
Hignett (1996b) UK	—	PO	PO	4.5
Johnston (1987) UK	7 student nurses	x-sect.	43%	3.5
Lagerström and Hagberg (1997) Sweden	348 nurses	quasi	76%	3.5
Nussbaum and Torres (2001) USA	24 female volunteers	quasi	59%	3.0
Raistrick (1981) UK	no information	survey	18%	2.0
Rodgers (1985b) UK	2 general medical and surgical wards (n = ?)	qual.	38%	3.5

Scopa (1993) USA	49 nurses	quasi	65%	4.0
Stubbs et al. (1983) UK	2 student nurses	quasi	55%	4.5
St Vincent et al. (1989) Canada	33 orderlies	x-sect.	70%	4.5
Troup and Rauhala (1987) UK and Finland	4 groups of student nurses	quasi	54%	3.0
Venning (1988) USA	—	PO	PO	4.0
Videman et al. (1989) Finland	200 student nurses	expt	41%	3.5
Wachs and Parker (1987) USA	178 nurses	x-sect.	86%	5.0
Wood (1987) Canada	nurses (n = ?)	quasi	56%	4.0

☺☺☺☺ Strong evidence from four high-quality studies (QR >75%) and eight moderate studies (QR 50–74%) that training interventions have no impact on working practices or injury rates

10.2 STUDIES DESCRIBING MIXED (POSITIVE AND NEGATIVE) RESULTS

The second section of this chapter has six studies which used experimental or quasi-experimental designs. They found mixed results with some positive effects after short-term or limited training intervention programmes.

Addington (1994)

This study investigated whether the number of reported back injuries, restricted working days and days off would drop following a back-care programme for operating room (OR) staff. The programme included shock-absorbing footwear, a fatigue-absorbing floor covering, body mechanics advice ('move, don't twist'), a fitness programme (stationary bicycles), a ten-week campaign and lumbar cushions. A twelve-month follow up looked at the number of incidents, number of restricted days and days off.

There was no decrease in the number of reported back injuries but there was a 60 per cent decrease in the number of restricted days/days off. Ninety per cent of staff were wearing the shock-absorbing footwear at the end of the twelve months, with positive feedback about the stationary bicycles. The study concluded that the purpose-designed programme had had an effect on sickness absence but not incidence rates.

Daws (1981)

This study used a training programme (half-day session, including a slide show).

Immediately after the programme started a reduction in back injuries was reported but twelve months later the injury rate was back to the pre-programme level.

Engels et al. (1998)

An investigation into whether postural load and ergonomic, biomechanical errors showed a decline following a training course based on theories of planned behaviour and concept of habitual behaviour. The intervention provided ten meetings to give training in safe practice and ergonomic awareness, and follow-up support meetings. The effect was measured by comparing four written protocols before the start of the course, three months after the course and fifteen months after. The subjects performed standardised tasks at these stages which were videoed and analysed using OWAS, RPE, checklist and time for task:

1   washing back and leg of a patient in bed;
2   bed–wheelchair transfer by lifting;
3   repositioning a patient up in bed; and
4   preparatory work, e.g. fetching towels, etc.

The results showed that the OWAS score and errors decreased significantly fifteen months after the course, especially for a lifting task (used hoist). However, the RPE increased, so new working behaviour did not lead to a decrease in perceived exertion.

Garrett and Perry (1996)

This paper described a cascade training programme which included movement and transfer techniques, therapeutic positioning, provision of back belts (worn by the carer) and the proper use of equipment with the intention of looking at the effect on lost-time injury cases. The intervention focused on three areas of high-risk tasks:

1   moving and turning patients in bed;
2   assisting patients to the standing position; and
3   transferring patients to/from bed.

Four rules were established:

1   if the patient is bigger than the carer, two people must assist;
2   exclusion criteria based on clinical contraindications;
3   two staff must assist in the transfer of all patients who are unable to help
     moving themselves up in bed; and
4   patients must wear trousers or pyjamas when transfer techniques are used.

Lost-time cases were evaluated over three years.

For nursing staff the number of lost-time cases reduced from forty-two to twenty-three cases per year, whereas therapy staff fluctuated from 2–0–3 over the three-year period. The authors concluded that the programme reduced injuries for nursing staff but not therapy staff.

Hellsing et al. (1993)

This study described the design, implementation and evaluation of an educational module within a nursing programme covering the prevention of back and neck pain by ergonomic and behavioural training. The programme was delivered as two hours of ergonomics tuition per week to include relaxation, physical and psychological training (including patient-transfer techniques), pain perception and stress management. It was supplemented by a three-day intensive course on patient transfers. The intervention and control groups were both evaluated at the start of the three years, half way through and one year after the end of the course using the Nordic Questionnaire, a non-standardised questionnaire about the educational package and observation, and PEO. Data were also collected for standardised work tasks, e.g. transfer bed–chair, making a bed, dressing a foot wound, taking a venous blood sample and distributing lunch.

The authors found that there were no obvious short-term effects of education on musculoskeletal problems, although the intervention group scored with respect to knowledge about body posture, psychosocial issues, work techniques and work factors. The observation data indicated that the control group tended to adopt more extreme postures (forward flexion) for longer times.

Lynch and Freund (2000)

This paper described a one-year back-injury training programme at a 440-bedded hospital. The training was delivered using a train-the-trainers programme and subsequent cascade sessions (1½ hour's duration) for nursing staff. A pre- and post-training questionnaire found that there was no change in the level of knowledge about back-injury risk factors. A change in work practices showing a reduction in the number of repositioning-in-bed tasks was reported for the trained group, although the authors suggested that this might have been due to avoidance of the task, with the control group carrying out the task. The reported lost-time back injuries showed a 30 per cent reduction on the average from the previous three years. It was concluded that training in the absence of engineering controls was inadequate to reduce back pain for departments with a high demand for patient handling.

Summary of evidence

Author and location	Subjects	Study type	QR	PR
Addington (1994) USA	operating-room staff (n = ?)	quasi	37%	3.0
Daws (1981) UK	2000 nursing staff	quasi	31%	2.5
Engels et al. (1998) Netherlands	24 licensed practical nurses	quasi	44%	3.0
Garrett and Perry (1996) USA	700 nurses	quasi	46%	3.5
Hellsing et al. (1993) Sweden	51 nursing students	expt	58%	3.5
Lynch and Freund (2000) USA	374 nurses	quasi	50%	3.5

☺☺☺ Moderate evidence from two studies that training interventions can have mixed (positive and negative), short-term results

10.3 STUDIES DESCRIBING POSITIVE OUTCOMES

The final section in this chapter includes nine studies which reported positive outcomes from predominantly training interventions. Again only one study (Scholey, 1983) has a high QR so the evidence level is moderate, rather than strong.

Alavosius and Sulzer-Azaroff (1986)

This study investigated the results of feedback on task performance and whether feedback improved safety when transferring patients. The carers were given written and verbal feedback on transfer safety initially on a weekly basis and subsequently at a longer interval (seven months). The intervention was evaluated using the percentage of safe transfers performed by each subject during baseline, feedback and follow-up conditions. Following feedback the safe performance of nearly all transfer components either improved or remained at high levels.

Best (1997)

This paper investigated the hypothesis that thirty-two hours' training in the manutention method of manual handling would decrease back strain and injuries in nurses working in geriatric care. The intervention was evaluated with:

1   postural analysis (OWAS);
2   a questionnaire about the frequency and severity of back pain;
3   RPE; and
4   nurses' perceptions of patient comfort and safety.

Over the twelve-month period no significant results were found for the postural analysis, RPE ratings or reported injuries, although all showed some improvement over the pre-intervention data.

Feldstein et al. (1993)

This evaluated an education programme in two hospitals which aimed to change nurses' behaviours. The programme was delivered on three shifts and included classroom instruction and eight hours of practical tuition to present information on body mechanics, techniques of patient transfer, one-on-one assistance, use of equipment, hazard identification and stretching/strengthening routines. The evaluation used a questionnaire before the intervention and one month later to look at body posture, transfer evaluation, flexibility test and proprioception tests.

Results showed that after the intervention the scores for composite back pain and composite fatigue went down for the intervention group (not statistically significant). A 19 per cent improvement in score was seen for the quality of patient transfers by the intervention group, which suggested that a short-term change in behaviour had been achieved.

Foster (1996)

This investigated the changes in nursing practice following the introduction of a manual-handling training programme based on the Scandinavian Back School. The change was evaluated using a self-completion questionnaire.

Results showed that there was a 74 per cent change in practice, with 77 per cent improved use of equipment. The author concluded that training had promoted positive changes in practice and equipment use; however, no control group or pre-/post-within-group information was provided.

Gray et al. (1996)

This lift-and-transfer education programme was based on Bobath Normal Movement concepts. It was delivered over five weeks with four hours on site per week and included: stretching (warm up); transfers; formal reading; repositioning; problem solving and equipment familiarisation. The knowledge of the lift and transfer procedures was tested using a quiz, and satisfaction with training was evaluated with a five-point scale.

The authors found that a significantly higher percentage of the intervention unit had correct answers compared with the control group.

Paternoster et al. (1999)

This study described a training intervention in an acute hospital. Eighty staff were given eight hours' training in theory and practice in three classroom sessions. Postural analysis data were collected by observation before and six months after the course (with different staff pre- and post-).

The study found that incorrect postures reduced from 68 per cent before the training to 38 per cent after the training. It was noted, however, that not using the same workers pre- and post- training led to an incorrect method of checking efficacy.

Scholey (1983)

This study investigated the null hypothesis that there would be no significant difference in truncal stress monitored before and after three weeks of training for three tasks:

1   turning a patient at night (rolling);
2   transfer bed–chair (pivot); and
3   transferring back to bed.

The outcome measures included IAP, observations to look at spinal posture and movement, techniques used, incidents causing sudden stress and interviews.

It was found that training reduced truncal stress for three of the four subjects, but the confounding factors were not controlled for this study (tasks were not identical even with the same patient).

Tuffnell (1989)

This study looked at the actions taken following a previous study which found that 289 lifts involved lifting most of the patient's weight. Intervention was a 'back-to-backs' programme which included three levels:

1   administrative: return-to-work programme, incident-reporting procedure and training programme at induction and two yearly refreshers;

2   charge nurses: identify lifting/team partners for each shift, nursing-care plans, review of equipment, warm-up exercises; and

3   individual level: warm up, plan lifts, work with partner, avoid drag lifts, report back symptoms.

Data were collected using self-reported questionnaires about the incidence of back pain, type of lifts and number of lifts performed over a shift.

After training it was found that more nurses were using the shoulder lift.

Wood et al. *(2000)*

This study described an intervention programme based on a training programme, information sheets, and SCOOT transfer which aimed to:

1   increase the most therapeutic weight bearing transfer technique to increase functional independence by decreasing the use of mechanical lifts and eliminating the two-person under-the-arm transfer through educating staff;

2   increase the accuracy of transfer information in bedside-care plans; and

3   decrease the number and cost of injuries to staff during transfers.

The programme was evaluated by:

1   checking the accuracy of the bedside information sheets;

2   employee-injury information; and

3   surveying staff transfer techniques (observation data).

It was found that only 37 per cent of bedside information sheets were accurate. Staff performed prescribed transfers 68 per cent of the time before the intervention; this rose to 92 per cent at a six-month follow-up. Similar improvements were seen with reminding residents not to hold the staff around the neck (36 per cent increased to 84 per cent), and the use of a mechanical lift transfer (10 per cent increased to 50 per cent). Injuries decreased from twenty-five to eleven, although this was still higher than the state-wide average. The authors concluded by saying that that individualised training on a small unit may be beneficial.

Summary of evidence

Author and location	Subjects	Study type	QR	PR
Alavosius and Sulzer-Azaroff (1986) USA	6 direct-care staff	quasi	39%	3.0
Best (1997) Australia	55 nursing and allied health staff at 3 nursing homes	quasi	70%	3.0

Feldstein *et al.* (1993) USA	55 nurses, aides and orderlies	quasi	68%	4.0
Foster (1996) UK	100 nurses	survey	57%	2.5
Gray *et al.* (1996) Canada	14 nursing units (n = ?)	quasi	43%	2.0
Paternoster *et al.* (1999) Italy	80 hospital workers	quasi	31%	2.0
Scholey (1983) UK	2 nurses, 2 student nurses	quasi	78%	2.0
Tuffnell (1989) New Zealand	nurses (n = ?)	survey	29.5%	1.5
Wood *et al.* (2000) USA	90 certified nursing assistants	quasi	46%	3.5

☺☺☺ Moderate evidence from four studies and limited evidence from four studies that intervention based on training can have short-term positive outcomes

CHAPTER 11

OTHER INTERVENTIONS

This chapter summarises the available research which describes interventions other than ones predominantly based on training (Chapter 10). The interventions have been grouped into four categories. Interventions which are:

1   based on, or including, risk assessment and management;
2   multi-factor interventions not based on risk management;
3   single-factor interventions (e.g. provision of equipment); and
4   lifting teams.

All four sections presented moderate evidence with at least two studies with a QR greater than 50 per cent. The multi-factor interventions (Sections 11.1 and 11.2) used many of the same strategies (e.g. equipment, training, policies, work-space redesign, etc.) but without staff involvement in the planning stages of the projects in Section 11.2.

Only two studies in Section 11.2 had a QR of over 50 per cent, with two others having a QR of 50 per cent. These are combined to give a moderate-evidence level statement. However there was also one high-quality study (>75 per cent) which found no significant difference between the pre- and post-intervention measures. This suggests that a multi-factor intervention based on risk assessment is more likely to be successful.

The use of a single-factor intervention is supported by two studies with a QR of greater than 75 per cent, giving a moderate-evidence level statement. Moderate evidence from three studies out of five suggests that interventions using the lifting-team approach are effective.

11.1 INTERVENTIONS BASED ON, OR INCLUDING, RISK MANAGEMENT

The largest number of studies are in the first section with nineteen studies included. Ten provide moderate evidence (QR score >50 per cent) that an intervention based on risk assessment shows benefits. This is supported by an additional four studies of lower quality. The outcome measures are wide ranging and some only show short-term results.

Alexander (1996)

This project evaluated a risk-management programme for community nurses with respect to the nursing managers' ability to implement the recommendations for risk reduction. The risk-reduction recommendations included the provision of hoists, increasing staffing levels, addressing space constraints, and tackling difficulties identified with both patients and carers (including sudden changes in clinical condition).

The author found that the managers perceived that an increased awareness through education would be the main factor in reducing sickness absence for back and neck pain whereas the staff believed that provision of equipment would be the main factor. A significant relationship was found with respect to implementation of risk-reduction recommendations and reduction in sickness absence. It was found to be three times lower (9 per cent compared with 28 per cent) in the implementation group than the non-implementation group over the twelve-month period.

Collins (1990)

This study examined an intervention which included a risk-management programme (injury-monitoring system, hazard registers, Back Injury Prevention Action Group, and patient-assessment system); education and training; and injury-management follow-up.

The author found a reduction in sickness absence from seventeen working days per claim to eleven working days per claim, but the injury rates fluctuated over the five-year period.

Duggan (1995)

This M.Sc. dissertation aimed to test whether the physical load on the musculo-skeletal system of nursing staff could be reduced by an ergonomic intervention. A multi-factor approach was used including:

1   equipment: adjustable-height bath, flat-access shower unit, raised patient lavatories, raised-height drug trolley, new bedside rails, new bath hoist, adjustable-height beds, replacement wheelchairs and commodes, handling belts and stools for feeding;
2   structural changes with respect to access and working space;
3   work organisation changes with respect to the bathing regime; and
4   an ergonomic educational programme including a patient-assessment system.

The intervention was evaluated using postural analysis (OWAS) for eighteen tasks and RPE for nineteen tasks.

The results highlighted a significant reduction in the harmful postures adopted post-intervention. The RPE results found that six of the tasks were no longer carried out post-intervention, and the remaining thirteen showed a significant reduction for the lower and upper back.

Evanoff et al. (1999)

This participatory ergonomics project was carried out with hospital orderlies to see if direct worker participation in problem solving would improve job satisfaction, injury rates, lost time and musculoskeletal symptoms. The participatory programme included an eight-hour training session for team building; provision of basic technical information about risk management; and regular meetings with supervisors and support group (doctor, occupational therapist and ergonomist).

As a result of the programme, two major factors were addressed:

- lack of standard procedures for lifting and handling patients; and
- inconsistent training procedures.

Changes included:

1 all manual lifts and transfers had to be done with two carers;
2 emphasis on the use of equipment (drawsheets, adjusting height of bed);
3 special procedures for heavy patients;
4 maintenance of equipment;
5 mirrors at busy intersections; and
6 evaluation of mechanical aids.

The intervention was evaluated using the OSHA 200 log, workers' compensation insurance records; self-administered surveys of workers at one, seven and fifteen months.

The authors found a decrease in risks of work injury, with a reduction in the relative risk of 50 per cent, for both OSHA 200 log and injury rate as well as a reduction in total days lost. The survey found a large and statistically significant reduction in the proportion of employees with musculoskeletal symptoms. The authors concluded by recommending the use of a participatory approach with a multi-factor intervention.

Fazel (1998)

This professional opinion described a programme to reduce the lost work time due to manual-handling-related accidents. An annual audit of manual-handling-related activity was undertaken which included a risk assessment of equipment, patient assessment and training, together with £100,000 being spent on patient-handling equipment (height adjustable baths, hoists, sliding sheets and inanimate load trolleys).

An 84 per cent reduction in lost hours was recorded in the second-year audit.

Fragala and Santamaria (1997)

This paper described an intervention over a three-year period which used a four-step approach:

1   risk identification and assessment;
2   risk analysis;
3   formulation of recommendations; and
4   implementation.

Through this process, involving all staff at the hospital, the two highest risk areas (orthopaedics and medical/surgical unit) were identified and patient lifting devices (a standing aid and hoist) were implemented. The implementation involved an educational awareness and training programme for the managers and nursing staff.

The results showed an overall reduction of 48 per cent in patient transfer incidents, a 67 per cent reduction in lost work days, and costs were reduced by 32 per cent in the first year and 44 per cent in the second year. The three key points from the programme were summarised as:

1   there must be a champion (individual or group) for the effect;
2   a system must be in place to design, implement and measure the impact of the programme; and
3   unacceptable high-risk job activities must be physically challenged.

Garg and Owen (1992)

This four-year ergonomic intervention in nursing homes aimed to reduce back stress. The intervention had six stages:

1   determination of patient-handling tasks perceived to be most stressful by nursing aides (NAs) (Owen and Garg, 1989; Garg et al., 1992);
2   ergonomic evaluation of the work performed by NAs prior to the introduction of change (Carlson, 1989);
3   pilot study to identify and locate assistive devices, to establish criteria for their selection and perform preliminary trials (Owen and Garg, 1990);
4   laboratory study on patient-handling devices (Garg et al., 1991 a and b);
5   intervention of selected devices into nursing homes and the training of NAs to use them with patients;
6   post-intervention measurement of back-injury incidence and severity rates, acceptability rates, biomechanical task demands and perceived level of physical stress.

Stages 5 and 6 are described in this paper. The following tasks were used for training: transfer bed–wheelchair; wheelchair–toilet; wheelchair–chairlift; in/out of bath tub; weighing patient. Hoists, walking belts with handles and a shower chair with removable foot pedals and arm supports were provided as additional equipment. The patients were classified as weight-bearing and dependent (using walking belt to transfer); dependent and non-weight-bearing (using hoist to transfer) and independent. The intervention was evaluated using acceptability rates (compliance with equipment assessed by observation); RPE; biomechanical evaluation; incidence of low-back pain; time for transfers; and number of NAs used in each transfer.

Overall there was an 81–96 per cent acceptance for the devices; the biomechanical stresses were significantly reduced (below the NIOSH action limit); the RPE for hoist and walking belt was reported as very, very light and very light; the injury rates fell from 83 per 200,000 work-hours lost to 47 per 200,000 work-hours lost. The authors concluded by saying that a systematic and appropriate ergonomic intervention could significantly reduce physical stresses to NAs and therefore reduce the future risk of musculoskeletal injuries.

Goodridge and Laurila (1997)

This quasi-experiment described the development, implementation and evaluation of a risk-management programme. The intervention was based on:

1   provision of patient-handling equipment (transfer belts, nylon sliders);
2   transfer-assessment tool;
3   training on equipment use; and
4   policies and procedures.

The programme was evaluated after two years by looking at records of staff injury rates. These fell from the baseline measure of 6.7 injuries per month to 4.1 injuries per month. The authors concluded that to be clinically effective the transfer-assessment tool had to be simple enough for the staff to easily incorporate it into practice, together with sufficient resources for equipment (and education on the use of the equipment).

Head and Levick (1996)

This study described the implementation of a no-lifting programme consisting of:

1   risk management;
2   hazard identification;
3   communication about the manual-handling initiative;
4   evaluation of equipment (beds, trolleys);
5   training;
6   policy; and
7   purchase of equipment.

The evaluation looked at the number of back-injury claims. The authors found a decrease in back injury claims, lost time and average cost in the first year. However, the authors questioned whether this decrease would be sustained as there appeared to be an increase after four years.

Hignett (2001b)

This paper gave retrospective information about a five-year ergonomics intervention programme which used a risk-management approach to tackle musculo-skeletal and manual-handling problems. The risk management was described as a top-down and bottom-up strategy including:

1   organisational policy;
2   risk assessments and audit programme;
3   participatory ergonomics projects (design decision groups);
4   product development;
5   building design;
6   equipment and furniture evaluation and purchase;
7   training (problem solving);
8   procedures; and
9   a patient-assessment system.

The results showed 36 per cent reduction in musculoskeletal sickness absence; 33 per cent reduction in manual-handling incidents; and an increase in completed risk actions from 33 to 76 per cent over the five years. The author recommended using an ergonomic approach with top-down and bottom-up strategies to embed ergonomics in the organisational culture.

Hignett and Richardson (1995)

This exploratory qualitative study looked at the perceptions of nursing staff towards manual-handling operations on the ward, including investigating the value of taking an ergonomic approach for risk management of handling human loads.

The findings proposed a new model for risk management to include the following factors:

1   patient;
2   worker;
3   workplace; and
4   organisational management interactions.

The authors recommended taking a structured approach to risk assessment based on a deeper understanding of the factors involved to address the problems and arrive at workable solutions, saying that tacit knowledge of experienced staff was not adequate for risk assessment.

Menckel et al. (1997)

Two strategies were evaluated for linking feedback directly to the taking of countermeasures:

1   feedback to all staff (work groups); and
2   written feedback to supervisors.

The intervention was evaluated by looking at the proposals produced for countermeasures. The authors found that although more proposals were generated by the work groups (all staff) more of the supervisor proposals were implemented. The work groups made more proposals for physical aids whereas the supervisors favoured training.

Miller and Johnson (1992)

This study set out to investigate whether having an appropriate risk assessment improved the working conditions for carers (home care). Three visits were made to assess the conditions and provide advice on:

1   handling and transferring;
2   time- and labour-saving techniques;
3   correct use and application of equipment; and
4   mobility at home and in the car.

The intervention was evaluated with a questionnaire.
    No improvement was found in carer general health, although confidence in using the techniques and equipment increased.

Mital and Shrey (1996)

This paper gave a professional opinion based on a review and critical appraisal of ergonomic studies of back problems in nursing.
    The authors recommended that an integrated approach of ergonomic intervention and a disability-management programme would reduce the inevitable back-injury record.

Monoghan et al. (1998)

This paper described the implementation of a no-lift policy. The policy was developed on six care-of-the-elderly wards, a day-hospital and an out-patient department. Initial brainstorming sessions were followed by a more formal risk-assessment programme which led to the identification of the proposed changes. These included the provision of equipment (two hoists and three adjustable-height plinths), training sessions and a patient-assessment form. Semi-structured questionnaires and the review of forty patient-care plans were used to evaluate the intervention. After nine months it was reported that 59 per cent of staff had attended training (which was considered to be disappointing) and 75 per cent of patients had mobility plans, but many had not been updated since admission. The authors concluded by saying that there had been a lack of multi-disciplinary collaboration.

Nyran (1991)

This study aimed to measure the direct costs of implementing the intervention programme in relation to the costs of patient-handling-related injuries among nursing personnel in nursing homes. A training programme was used which included a two-day course (including ergonomic risk assessment) with a five-hour follow up at six months. Actions from the risk assessments were implemented during the intervention including: purchase of hoists; variable-height beds; new wheelchairs with detachable arm/leg rests; and equipment maintenance. The intervention was evaluated using:

1   injury status eight months prior to the training, and eight months after;
2   lost-time claims from the compensation board; and
3   additional data from interviews with senior and middle managers before and after the training.

The results showed that there was a net saving of $57,440 (saving in lost-time injuries, including the cost of the training) in four out of the five nursing homes. The conclusion was that intensive training had some impact on the reduction in the number of workers' compensation board claims. The interviews suggested that there was a reduction in the severity of the cases.

Peers (1998)

This intervention used were:

1   risk assessments;
2   individual bedside logos for correct method of transfer;
3   assessment of every resident before lift/transfer;
4   an education programme; and
5   the provision of sliding sheets for repositioning in bed.

The evaluation looked at lost time and the number of staff on decreased work capacity. There was a reduction in lost time and number of staff on modified duties.

Pohjonen et al. (1998)

This study investigated the effects and feasibility of a twelve-month ergonomic intervention on work content and load in home-care work included measures which were designed and implemented as part of a participatory approach based on team work and group problem solving within the work unit. The interventions included:

1   group problem solving;
2   changing/redesigning the equipment used;
3   purchase of new equipment;
4   changing the methods for using equipment;
5   increasing the possibilities for regulating the work pace; and
6   discussing the goals of the work with the clients.

Work-site assessments included questionnaires (including WAI), work-sampling study, work-physiological measurements (heart-rate monitor) and postural analysis (OWAS).

The authors found that the proportion of straight-back positions increased significantly due to the intervention (from 59 to 75 per cent). Subjects were better able to utilise their own abilities and needs to adjust the work rate as a result of the intervention. The ergonomic measures improved both physical and mental work content and working conditions and prevented the decline of work ability in the intervention group. The conclusion was that participatory ergonomics was an effective and feasible way of reducing the workload and increasing the job satisfaction of ageing female home-care workers.

Tracy (1996)

This professional opinion described an intervention programme which sought to reduce manual-handling incidents over a four-year period. The intervention was based on risk assessment and included the introduction of a no-lifting policy and provision of equipment (hoists and height-adjustable baths). A trend showing a reduction in incident reports was described which was attributed to the intervention programme.

Summary of evidence

Author and location	Subjects	Study type	QR	PR
Alexander (1996) UK	42 community nurse managers, 93 community nurses	survey	50%	5.0
Collins (1990) Australia	nurses (n = ?)	quasi	52%	5.0

Duggan (1995) Ireland	20 nursing staff on geriatric ward	quasi	74%	5.0
Evanoff et al. (1999) USA	67 hospital orderlies	quasi	58%	5.0
Fazel (1998) UK	hospital staff (no detail)	PO	PO	4.0
Fragala and Santamaria (1997) USA	1 hospital (no detail)	PO	PO	4.0
Garg and Owen (1992) USA	57 nursing assistants	quasi	63%	5.0
Goodridge and Laurila (1997) Canada	nurses (n = ?)	quasi	44%	3.5
Head and Levick (1996) Australia	nurses and ambulance personnel (n = ?)	quasi	28%	3.5
Hignett (2001b) UK	5000 hospital staff	PO	PO	4.5
Hignett and Richardson (1995) UK	26 nurses	qual.	81%	4.5
Menckel et al. (1997) Sweden	122 health-care staff	quasi	63%	4.0
Miller and Johnson (1992) UK	10 carers	survey	50%	3.5
Mital and Shrey (1996) USA	—	PO	PO	4.5
Monoghan et al. (1998) UK	28 staff	quasi	31%	2.5
Nyran (1991) Canada	48 nursing personnel	case	65%	4.0
Peers (1998) Canada	131 nursing-home staff	quasi	37%	3.0

Pohjonen et al. (1998) Finland	70 home-care workers	expt	58%	4.5
Tracy (1996) UK	2400 hospital staff	PO	PO	4.0

☺☺☺ Moderate evidence from ten studies with QR scores ≥50% and an additional four studies with QR scores between 25% and 49% that interventions should be based on risk assessment

☺☺☺ Moderate evidence from two studies that managers and supervisors tend to support a training/education intervention whereas staff support the provision of physical aids (equipment)

11.2 MULTI-FACTOR INTERVENTIONS NOT BASED ON RISK ASSESSMENT

The second section has ten studies showing mixed findings. These studies are mostly based on expert advisors (steering groups) putting forward a planned intervention rather than the intervention strategy arising from the staff through a risk-management process. Several lower-quality studies reported positive findings with decreases in sickness absence or lifting load due to multi-factor interventions, but two studies reported no change in their outcome measures.

Aird (1988)

This pilot project assessed the effectiveness of an ergonomics programme for back-injury prevention. Two cases were described in a hospital and a home for the aged. The hospital programme included:

1   medical examination at induction and return to work;
2   assessment of lifting skills;
3   monthly education on back care and lifting;
4   job training and problem-solving sessions; and
5   a general fitness programme.

The home-for-the-aged programme included:

1   back-care education;
2   mechanical aids;
3   detailed patient assessment; and
4   regular education sessions.

The programme was evaluated using lost-time-injury claim information for strain and sprain injuries by occupational group and body part.

The hospital case study reported a reduction in back injuries by 8.4 per cent and in frequency by 18.8 per cent. The home for the aged reported no back injuries in the twelve months following the start of the intervention. The study concluded that the pilot project provided preliminary support for the effectiveness of a multi-faceted ergonomic approach to back-injury prevention.

Daynard et al. (2001)

A comparison of two strategies:

1   improved patient-handling technique with existing equipment; and
2   improved patient-handling technique with new assistive and mechanical equipment; against
3   a control group.

The comparison was based on peak and cumulative spinal compression and reaction shear at L4/5 during a series of simulated patient-handling activities using light/cooperative (55 kg) and heavy/passive (100 kg) patients:

1   bed-to-wheelchair transfer (light patient with standing hoist; transfer belt pivot with two carers; heavy patient with hoist);
2   bed-to-stretcher transfer (slide board, padded and non-padded tube sliding sheets with two to three carers, sliding sheet with three carers);
3   bed boost (padded tube sliding sheet with three carers, sliding sheet with two carers);
4   chair boost (transfer belt with two carers, transfer belt with one carer, sliding sheet with two carers, hoist);
5   bed turn (padded tube sliding sheet with two carers, sliding sheet with two carers).

A biomechanical assessment and analysis were done using WATBAK for peak and cumulative compressive and shear loads at L4/5. Data were collected using a video and hand-force dynamometer. Compliance was assessed with respect to the training received.

The authors found that compliance was significantly greater with the heavy patient in all activities except for the bed–stretcher transfer. The training-only group (1) was compliant less than 50 per cent of the time whereas the training with equipment group (2) had increased compliance by 20 per cent and had reduced spinal loading in several tasks. The time taken in all but the bed–stretcher transfer was significantly longer when equipment was used. The bed–wheelchair and chair-boost activities generated peak spinal compressions exceeding the NIOSH limit, although this reduced with the use of equipment. The use of assistive devices was associated with significantly greater cumulative spinal loads and reaction shear than manual transfer. This indicated that the use of equipment decreased the peak spinal compression but increased the cumulative spinal load and reaction shear. The authors suggested that this was mostly likely due to the increased number of push/pull forces and the increased time in a forward flexion position while preparing the patient.

Dixon et al. (1996)

This study described the implementation of a no-lifting standard which aimed to stop the manual lifting of patients and reduce the risk of injury to nurses. The standard set out that:

1   no lifting of patients should occur except in exceptional circumstances (cardiac or respiratory arrest with patient on the floor; unconscious patient on the floor, fall in a confined area, post-total-hip replacement, patient on floor with suspected fractured spine, hips or legs, evacuation for fire), where procedures were in place;
2   equipment was provided (hoist with extra slings, lateral transfer board, roller board, turntables); and
3   one-to-one training was provided for all staff.

The implementation was evaluated using staff sickness resulting from back injury.

No episodes of staff sickness were reported following implementation. Subjective reports from staff suggested that they were more able to cope with the physical demands of work and were less tired at the end of a shift.

Entwhistle et al. (1996)

This intervention programme included:

1   the assessment of patient-handling requirements and the provision of hoists/equipment where needed;
2   an improvement in educational literature and lifting training;
3   the development of a lifting policy, code of practice and performance standard for lifting;
4   patient-handling assessment form and care plan; and
5   a review of uniforms and other practical requirements for safe lifting (culottes and trousers).

Evaluation was through the:

1   episodes of certificated illness associated with back pain;
2   training attendance;
3   customer survey questionnaire.

The number of certificated episodes reduced from thirty-five in the previous year to eight episodes in the first six months of the intervention. Attitudes were reported to have changed, with 93 per cent saying they had changed their handling practices.

Kilbom et al. (1985)

This cross-sectional study evaluated the effect of modern equipment, improved workspace design and work organisation. A traditional ward, with cramped conditions and a few out-of-date hoists, was compared to a modern ward with spacious rooms and adequate equipment. The outcome measures included a strain gauge to calculate the vertical force, the duration of the lift and the weight distribution between feet to calculate symmetry.

Results showed that the total weight, the number of lifts with asymmetry and the duration of the lifts were lower in the modern ward. The authors concluded by saying that the strain due to lifting in geriatric care could be reduced with the aid of modern hoists and well designed spacious wards.

Ljungberg et al. (1989)

This study compared work loads in an old-style ward with a more modern-style ward by assessing work time; lifts per hour; average load; lift duration; weight distribution during lift; OWAS; physiological function; handling-needs score for patients; and RPE.

Results showed that lifting work was approximately 50 per cent less in the modern ward which had:

1   easily manoeuvred electric overhead hoists;
2   spacious premises; and
3   better work organisation, although the patient-handling needs were equiva-
     lent.

The authors recommended that older or under-equipped wards should possibly be compensated in the form of extra staff; hoists should be used to prepare for unforeseen incidents; and adequate space should be provided with respect to beds, doorways and toilets.

Oddy (1993)

This six-month programme aimed to reduce manual lifting to an absolute minimum and to encourage as many patients on a continuing-care ward of twenty-four patients as possible to bear weight through their feet while being helped to move with dignity and safety. The intervention included:

1   handling guidance in care plans;
2   replanning the layout of the ward to include additional hand rails, adjusting
     the height of existing hand rails; and

3   reviewing the suitability of seating for nursing access as well as patient comfort.

The intervention was evaluated based on the elimination of the lug/drag method of lifting. Results showed the reduction over the six months of the lug/drag method with alternative methods being used instead (pivot transfer, hoist, assisted transfer, and walking with two carers). It was suggested that the success of the project was due to the willingness of the nursing staff to make the changes, the monitoring of the wards by the nursing supervisor, and the collaborative approach to training.

Torri et al. (1999)

The third and fifth phases of this multi-factor management of risk procedure are relevant to this review. The authors described a survey and analysis of sickness absence due to low-back pain and an assessment of the preventative interventions (staff training and the introduction of equipment) included in the study. The outcome measures included sickness absence and a questionnaire on hoist use.

The results showed a 39 per cent reduction in sickness absence due to low-back pain between 1995 and 1997 and that 71 per cent of staff used the hoists regularly and correctly.

Tracz and Rose (1982)

This retrospective analysis of an intervention was based on the introduction of equipment and training on a thirty-bedded rehabilitation ward. The intervention included:

1   weekly lectures from physiotherapists on body mechanics and lifting and individual patient assessment;
2   mechanical lifts (hoists);
3   safety inspection of ward; and
4   occupational health assessment for individual staff.

The impact was measured by the number of reported injuries and time lost for back-related injuries.

The authors found that there was little change following the remedial actions and reported that they believed that there was a greater reduction in the time lost by increasing the staffing levels.

Trevelyan (2001)

This study described the findings of an ergonomic intervention and the methods used to evaluate exposure. The intervention included:

1   a relaunch of the manual-handling policy;

2   work organisational initiatives with link-nurse scheme;
3   provision of equipment (high–low baths, hoists; transfer belts; sliding sheets); and
4   on-site training (two-day programme).

The evaluation of the intervention used:

1   self-reported questionnaire about health, frequency of tasks, posture, use of equipment and psychosocial factors;
2   task analysis; and
3   PEO.

Results from the questionnaire and task analysis showed no significant differences pre/post intervention and the PEO results were limited due to within-task variability.

Summary of evidence

Author and location	Subjects	Study type	QR	PR
Aird (1988) Canada	3 hospitals (n = ?)	case	44%	4.0
Daynard et al. (2001) Canada	36 unit assistants	quasi	81%	5.0
Dixon et al. (1996) UK	27-bed mixed elderly-care medical ward	quasi	20%	3.0
Entwhistle et al. (1996) UK	nurses (n = 900)	quasi	35%	3.0
Kilbom et al. (1985) Sweden	12 nurses	x-sect.	27%	3.0
Ljungberg et al. (1989) Sweden	24 nursing aides	quasi	65%	4.0
Oddy (1993) UK	nurses (n = 24)	quasi	50%	3.5
Torri et al. (1999) Italy	all staff at 2 hospitals (approx. 900 staff)	quasi	50%	4.0
Tracz and Rose (1982) Canada	staff on 30-bed rehabilitation ward	quasi	33%	4.0
Trevelyan (2001) UK	48 nurses	quasi	78%	4.0

☺☺☺   Moderate evidence from three studies that multi-factor interventions can
show improvements. Contradictory evidence from one high-quality study
shows no improvement using a multi-factor intervention

11.3 SINGLE-FACTOR INTERVENTIONS

The third section includes six studies based on single intervention factors. These
included the use of back belts (worn by the carer), provision of a wide range of
moving and handling equipment; provision of sling hoists and standing-assist
hoists; and the accessibility/availability of handling aids. One of the studies has a
high QR (>75 per cent) with respect to the use of lifting (hoisting) equipment with
one other study having a QR of 52 per cent, so the evidence level is moderate.

Allen and Wilder (1996)

The effect of using a back belt on back-injury incident rates was evaluated by
training control and experimental groups in biomechanics and lifting techniques,
with the experimental group being asked to wear back belts when they were
lifting patients. The incident rate was calculated from the total number of incidents, total hours worked and total hours lost over a six-month period.

Results showed a significant difference between the control (three incidents)
and experimental (no incidents) group. The authors concluded that using back
belts in addition to education reduces injury-incident rate at least in the short term.

Duffy et al. (1999)

This team investigated the availability/accessibility of handling aids with respect
to their frequency of use and the amount of training received. They collected
data using a questionnaire. The results showed that all wards had at least one
type of handling aid but that most were underused (no aid used for 66 per cent
of manual-handling activities). Training on handling aids varied from three
minutes to two hours (average nineteen minutes). The most commonly found aid
was a handling sling (93 per cent) followed by hoists (73 per cent) and handling
belts (13 per cent). The authors suggested that aids should be more available
with training provided to facilitate use.

Fourie et al. (1992)

This study looked at independent bridging by patients with a fractured pelvis to
compare the provision of written instructions above patients' beds with respect
to pillow positioning (to bring shoulders higher than buttocks) and the use of a
lifting pole.

The authors found that the experimental group achieved independent bridging earlier. This facilitated the use of bed pans and functional use of hip muscles.

Fragala (1993)

This intervention assessed the potential worth of a mechanical-lift-based ergonomics system to reduce workplace back injuries. It used a sling lift (hoist) for total transfers and a standing assist lift (standing hoist) to replace manual stand-and-pivot transfers. The two-month pilot intervention study was evaluated with a questionnaire and a review of incident reports.

The author found that during the trial there were two incident reports, and an additional eight in the nine months following the trial compared with twelve in the previous calendar year. No conclusion was reported.

Holliday et al. (1994)

This pilot study looked at the impact of the introduction of new mechanical-lift technology in two long-term nursing units. The use of a new overhead system was compared with an old-style wheeled mechanical hoist. The outcome, measures included number of staff required for a lift, time taken, RPE and patient-comfort rating.

The results showed that fewer staff were required for the new system, RPE was significantly less but that there was no difference in comfort or time taken.

Knibbe and Friele (1999)

This intervention included the provision of forty patient hoists being introduced over a twelve-month period in 139 nursing homes and compared with 239 control nursing homes, with training, ergonomic assessment forms and lifting coordinators. The outcome measures included RPE, general epidemiological information and a specifically-designed recording tool (Log). Log has eleven categories to record the nursing activity relating to patient transfer; three options for patient cooperation; number of carers involved; assistance from informal care; use of equipment; and patient weight.

The authors found that the twelve-month back pain prevalence was reduced significantly in the intervention group, whereas the control group showed no change. The Log showed a decrease in the exposure for wheelchair transfers, bed transfers, and showering (sitting). The conclusion was that hoists provided a solution for approximately 33 per cent of the total number of transfers. The intervention group had a reduction in transfers for both hoist (50 per cent) and non-hoist (35 per cent) transfers, with no change in the control group. At the end of the intervention all passive patients in the intervention group were lifted with a hoist (compared with 67 per cent at the start).

Summary of evidence

Author and location	Subjects	Study type	QR	PR
Allen and Wilder (1996) USA	47 nurses	quasi	52%	2.5
Duffy et al. (1999) Ireland	150 nurses	survey	39%	3.0
Fourie et al. (1992) South Africa	80 patients	quasi	85%	5.0
Fragala (1993) USA	ward staff (n = ?)	quasi	46%	3.0
Holliday et al. (1994) Canada	22 nurses	quasi	50%	4.5
Knibbe and Friele (1999) Netherlands	378 home-care nurses	quasi	83%	5.0

☺☺☺ Moderate evidence from two studies that single-factor interventions based on the provision of equipment can be effective

☺☺ Limited evidence from one study that back belts (with education) can reduce injury rates in the short term

☺☺ Limited evidence from one study that written instructions about pillow positioning at the bedside can facilitate earlier independent bridging

11.4 LIFTING TEAM

The final section (11.4) reports five studies on interventions based on the use of lifting teams. Three of the studies have a quality rating of >50 per cent, so there is moderate evidence that an intervention based on a lifting-team approach is effective.

Caska et al. (1998)

This pilot study looked at the impact of a nurse-staffed lift team on a unit through the reallocation of existing staff in a 400-bed medical centre. The lift team comprised four staff and had a baseline standard of two-carer transfers with additional help from ward staff if required. The programme was evaluated by looking at:

1   the ability of the lift team to meet the demands for performance of patient transfers;

2   a survey on nursing reactions to the lift team;

3   injuries incurred from compensation records;

4   daily logs of transfer location and type, equipment used; and

5   whether the transfer was successful.

Results showed that the lift team completed 94 per cent of scheduled and paged lifts. Ninety-one per cent of nursing staff believed that the team should be continued after the pilot. No musculoskeletal discomfort or pain was recorded by the lift team. The transfer belt was the commonly-used equipment (71 per cent of transfers). The study concluded by saying that it was feasible to create an effective and frequently used lift team through reallocation of existing nursing staff members.

Charney (1997)

This paper described a series of interventions at ten hospitals (nine acute, one long care) using lifting teams for varying durations. The interventions were evaluated using OSHA 200 logs to calculate the injury rates for long-time injury, days lost and incidence rate, questionnaires looking at nurse satisfaction, and data on the compensation costs saved.

All ten facilities showed decreases in the number of nursing personnel with back injuries due to patient lifting (mean reduction in incident rates of 62.5 per cent and lost work-days of 90 per cent). Nursing satisfaction was found to be excellent. Facilities were found to average fifty lifts per shift (for 300-bed hospital).

Charney et al. (1991)

This pilot study investigated whether reducing by 95 per cent the number of lifts performed by nurses would result in a 95 per cent reduction in lost-time back injuries due to lifting patients. Ward orderlies were recruited onto a lifting team. Accident data were compared pre- and post-intervention.

Results showed a reduction in nursing sick leave, and that the lifting team had no sick leave. A saving was recorded on labour costs both for staff (orderlies were cheaper) and a reduction in compensation payments.

Charney et al. (1993)

This study is the same as Charney et al. (1991), with additional data for the second year of the intervention approach using a lifting team.

Year one saw a reduction from sixteen accidents per year to one, year two had no recorded accidents. The authors calculated that the lifting team had saved $65,000 over the twelve months for the day shift. The lifting team response time was five minutes. The conclusion was that a 350–400-bed facility could be lifted by two staff teams as only 8–12 per cent of patients were lifted during the course of the study year.

Santora (editorial) (1994)

This editorial described an intervention using a lifting team at a 65-bed neurological floor for six months. Members of the lifting team were selected based on their ability to lift 50–75 lbs frequently and more than 100 lbs occasionally, although hoists and slide boards were used as well.

Results showed that the lifting team handled 90 per cent of the lifts which led to a 90 per cent reduction in back injuries in nursing personnel.

Summary of evidence

Author and location	Subjects	Study type	QR	PR
Caska et al. (1998) USA	4 staff on lift team at 400-bed medical centre	quasi	69%	4.0
Charney (1997) USA	hospital staff at 10 hospitals	quasi	72%	4.0
Charney et al. (1991) USA	2 orderlies on lift team	quasi	37%	2.0
Charney et al. (1993) USA	orderlies on lift team (n = ?)	quasi	61%	3.5
Santoro (editorial) (1994) USA	65-bed neurology floor staff	quasi	35%	2.5

☺☺☺ Moderate evidence from three studies that interventions using the lifting-team approach can be effective

REFERENCES

Addington, C. (1994) 'All the right moves. A program to reduce back injuries in OR nurses', *AORN Journal* 59 (2): 483–8.

Aird, J.W. (1988) 'Comprehensive back injury prevention programme: an ergonomic approach for controlling back injuries in health care facilities', in Aghazadeh, F. (ed.) *Trends in Ergonomics Human Factors* V, Elsevier Science Publishers B.V., 705–12.

Alavosius, M.P. and Sulzer-Azaroff, B. (1986) 'The effects of performance feedback on the safety of client lifting and transfer', *Journal of Applied Behaviour Analysis* 19 (3): 261–7.

Alexander, P. (1998) 'Risk management in manual handling for community nurses', in Hanson, M. (ed.) (1988) *Contemporary Ergonomics,* 87–91.

Allen, S.K. and Wilder, K. (1996) 'Back belts pay off for nurses', *Occupational Health & Safety* 65: 59–62.

ASSTSAS (1999) *Principles for Moving Patients Safely,* L'Association pour la santé et la sécurité du travail, secteur affaires socials (ASSTSAS), Canada: Montréal.

Atkinson, F.I. (1992) 'Experiences of informal carers providing nursing support for disabled dependants', *Journal of Advanced Nursing* 17: 835–40.

Baglioni, A. (1999) 'Environmental features of hospital wards and interaction with patient handling', *Giornale Italiano di Medicina del Lavoro* 90 (2): 141–51.

Ballard, J. (1994) 'District nurses – who's looking after them?' *Occupational Health Review* November/December 10–16.

Bell, F. (1984) *Patient-Listing Devices in Hospitals,* London: Croom Helm, 120–209.

Bell, F. (1987) 'Ergonomic aspects of equipment', *International Journal of Nursing Studies* 24 (4): 331–7.

Bell, F., Dalgity, M.E., Fennell, M.J. and Aitken, R.C.B. (1979*)* 'Hospital ward patient-lifting tasks', *Ergonomics* 22 (11): 1257–73.

Benevolo, E., Sessarego, P., Zelaschi, G. and Franchignoni. F. (1993) 'An ergonomic analysis of five techniques for moving patients', *Giornale Italiano di Medicina del Lavoro* 15: 139–44.

Bernard, B.P. (ed.) (1997) 'Musculoskeletal disorders and work place factors. A critical review of epidemiologic for work-related musculoskeletal disorders of the neck, upper extremities and low back', *NIOSH: US Department of Health and Human Sciences,* 1.13–1.14.

Bertolazzi, M. and Saia, B. (1999) 'Risk during manual movement of loads', *Giornale Italiano di Medicina del Lavoro* 21 (2): 130–3.

Best, M. (1997) 'An evaluation of manutention training in preventing back strain and resultant injuries in nurses', *Safety Science* 25 (1–3): 207–22.

Bewick, N. and Gardner, D. (2000) 'Manual handling injuries in health care workers', *International Journal of Occupational Safety and Ergonomics* 6 (2): 209–21.

Billin, S.L. (1998) 'Moving and handing practice in neuro-disability nursing', *British Journal of Nursing* 7 (10): 571–8.

Billin, S.L. (2001) 'Safer handling practice in a neuro-disability environment', *The Column* 13 (1): 25–7.

Botha, W.E. and Bridger, R.S. (1998) 'Anthropometric variability, equipment usability and musculoskeletal pain in a group of nurses in the Western Cape', *Applied Ergonomics* 29 (6): 481–90.

Brulin, C., Winkvist, A. and Langendoen, S. (2000) 'Stress from working conditions among home care personnel with musculoskeletal symptoms', *Journal of Advanced Nursing* 31 (1): 181–9.

Bruno, C. and Davis, T. (1997) 'Redesign of the standard hospital wheelchair', in Sprigle, S. (ed.) *Proceedings of the RESNA 1997 Annual Conference, Pittsburgh, Pennsylvania,* Arlington, Virginia: RESNA Press, 75–7.

Busse, M. (2000) 'Effective rehabilitation and hoisting equipment: a case study', *Nursing & Residential Care* 2 (4): 168–73.

Caboor, D., Verlinden, M., Zinzen, E., Van Roy, P., Van Riel, M.P. and Clarys, J.P. (2000) 'Implications of an adjustable bed height during standard nursing tasks on spinal motion, perceived exertion and muscular activity', *Ergonomics* 43 (10): 1771–80.

Cameron, I., Crotty, M., Currie, C., Finnegan, T., Gillespie, L. and Gillespie W. (2000) 'Geriatric rehabilitation following fractures in older people: a systematic review', *Health Technol Assess* 4 (2).

Carlson, B.L. (1989) 'Ergonomic job evaluation of nursing assistants at Rock County health care nursing home facility', M.S. Thesis, Dept. of Industrial and Systems Engineering, University of Wisconsin, Milwaukee, WI. cited in Garg, A., Owen, B., Beller, D., and Banaag, J.A., (1991a) 'Biomechanical and ergonomic evaluation of patient transferring tasks: bed to wheelchair and wheelchair to bed', *Ergonomics* 34 (3): 289–312.

Caska, B.A., Patnode, R.E. and Clickner, D. (1998) 'Feasibility of a nurse staffed lift team', *AAOHN Journal* 46 (6): 283–8.

Chalmers, I. and Altman, D.G. (eds) (1995) *Systematic Reviews,* London: BMJ Publishing Group.

Charney, W. (1997) 'The lift team method for reducing back injuries: A 10 hospital study', *AAOHN Journal* 45 (6): 300–4.

Charney, W., Zimmerman, K. and Walara, E. (1991) 'The lifting team. A design method to reduce lost time back injury in nursing', *AAOHN Journal* 39: 231–4.

Charney, W., Zimmerman, K. and Walara, E. (1993) 'A design method to reduce lost time back injury in nursing' in Charney, W. and Schirmer, J. *Essentials of Modern Hospital Safety:2,* Lewis Publishers, 313–24.

Chartered Society of Physiotherapy (1998) 'Moving and handling for chartered physiotherapists', London: Chartered Society of Physiotherapy.

Coleman, S. and Brooke, S. (1999) 'Manual handling in the operating theatre', *Professional Nurse* 14 (10): 682–6.

Collins, B. (1994) 'Objective manual material handling assessments in the ambulance service using the lumbar monitor industrial package', *Ambulance* 9: 10–14.

Collins, B. (1998) 'Back supports as part of an integrated programme of back injury prevention in the ambulance service', *Ambulance UK* 13 (6): 281–4.

Collins, M. (1990) 'A comprehensive approach to preventing occupational back pain among nurses', *Journal of Occupational Health & Safety – Australia & New Zealand* 6 (5): 361–8.

Conneeley, A.L. (1992) 'The impact of the manual handling operations regulations on the use of hoists in the home: the patient's perspective', *British Journal of Occupational Therapy* 61 (1): 17–21.

Connolly, M.J., Wilkinson, E., Flanagan, S. and Mulley, G.P. (1990) 'Nurses' attitudes to and use of patient hoists in hospital', *Clinical Rehabilitation* 4: 13–17.

Corlett, E.N., Lloyd, P.V., Tarling, C., Troup, J.D.G. and Wright, B. (1992) *The Guide to the Handling of Patients* (3rd edn) National Back Pain Association/Royal College of Nursing.

CRD (2000) 'Undertaking systematic reviews of research on effectiveness', *CRD's Guidance for Carrying Out or Commissioning Reviews*: CRD Report 4, (draft), http://www.york.ac.uk/inst/crd/report4.htm.

Crumpton, E., Hignett, S., Goodwin, R. and Dewey, M. (2002) 'Reliability study of a data extraction and quality assurance tool applied to literature on patient handling', in P.T. McCabe (ed.) *Contemporary Ergonomics 2002*, London: Taylor & Francis, 51–6.

CSP (1975) *Handling the Handicapped. A Guide to the Lifting and Movement of Disabled People*, Cambridge: Woodhead-Faulkner Ltd.

Daws, J. (1981) 'Lifting and moving patients 3. A revision training programme', *Nursing Times*, November 25: 2067–9.

Daynard, D., Yassi, A., Cooper, J.E., Tate, R., Norman, R. and Wells, R. (2001) 'Biomechanical analysis of peak and cumulative spinal loads during simulated patient-handling activities: a substudy of a randomised controlled trial to prevent lift and transfer injury of health care workers', *Applied Ergonomics* 32: 199–214.

De Looze, M.P., Zinzen, E., Caboor, D., Heyblom, P., Van Bree, E., Van Roy, P. Toussaint, H.M. and Clarijs, J.P. (1994) 'Effect of individually chosen bed-height adjustments on the low-back stress of nurses', *Scandinavian Journal of Work, Environment & Health* 20: 427–34.

De Looze, M.P., Zinzen, E., Caboor, D. Van Roy, P., and Clarijs, J.P. (1988) 'Muscle strength, task performance and low back load in nurses', *Ergonomics* 41 (8): 1095–104.

DeGeorge, P. and Dunwoody, C. (1995) 'Transfer techniques of the lower extremity with an external fixator', *Orthopaedic Nursing* 14: 17–21.

Dehlin, O., and Lindberg, B. (1975) 'Lifting burden for a nursing aide during patient care in a geriatric ward', *Scandinavian Journal of Rehabilitation Medicine* 7: 65–72.

Dehlin, O. Hedenrud, B. and Horal, J. (1976) 'Back symptoms in nursing aides in a geriatric hospital. An interview study with special reference to the incidence of low-back symptoms', *Scandinavian Journal of Rehabilitation Medicine* 8: 47–53.

Derbyshire Interagency Group (2001) *Care handling for people in hospital, community and educational settings. A code of practice*, Southern Derbyshire NHS Trust (Community Health), North Derbyshire NHS Trust (Community Health), Derbyshire County Council Social Services, Derbyshire Local Educational Authority, Derbyshire Royal Hospital NHS Trust, Southern Derbyshire Acute Hospitals NHS Trust.

Dhoot, R. and Georgieva, C. (1996) 'The evolution bed in the NHS hospital environment', unpublished report, Lancaster University: The Management School.

Dietz, E. and Baumann, M. (2000) 'Obstacles to change: discussion and points of view of health care professionals with regard to the application patient-handling training', *Archives des Maladies Professionnelles et de Medecine du Travail* 61 (6): 389–95.

Disabled Living Foundation (2001) *Handling People: Equipment, Advice and Information* (2nd edn), London: Disabled Living Foundation.

Dixon, R., Lloyd, B. and Coleman, S. (1996) 'Defining and implementing a no lifting standard', *Nursing Standard* 10 (44): 33–6.

Dolan, P., Standell, C.J., Adams, G.G., Mannion, A.F. and Adams M.A. (1998) 'Spinal loading during manual handling procedures in nursing', *Proceedings of the International Society for the Study of the Lumbar Spine*, Belgium: Brussels, 80.

Doormaal, M., Driessen, A., Landeweerd, J. and Drost, M.R. (1995) 'Physical workload of ambulance assistants', *Ergonomics* 38 (2): 361–76.

Downs, S.H. and Black, N. (1998) 'The feasibility of creating a checklist for the assessment of the methodological quality both of randomised and non-randomised studies of health care interventions', *Journal of Epidemiological Community Health* 52: 377–84.

Duffy, A., Burke, C. and Dockrell, S. (1999) 'The use of lifting and handling aids by hospital nurses', *British Journal of Therapy and Rehabilitation* 6 (1): 20–4.

Duggan, E.A. (1995) 'An ergonomics approach to the reduction of the physical load of some nurses', unpublished M.Sc. dissertation, University of Limerick.

Edlund, C.K., Harms-Ringdahl, K. and Ekholm, J. (1998) 'Properties of person hoist spreader bars and their influence on sitting/lifting position', *Scandinavian Journal of Rehabilitation Medicine* 30 (3): 151–8.

Elford, W., Straker, L. and Strauss, G. (2000) 'Patient handling with and without slings: an analysis of the risk of injury to the lumbar spine', *Applied Ergonomics* 31: 185–200.

Ellis, B.E. (1993) 'Moving and handling patients: An evaluation of current training for physiotherapy students', *Physiotherapy* 79: 323–6.

Engels, J.A., Landeweerd, J.A. and Kant, Y. (1994) 'An OWAS based analysis of nurses' working postures', *Ergonomics* 37: 909–19.

Engels, J.A., van der Gulden, J.W., Senden, T.F., Kolk, J.J. and Binkhorst, R.A. (1998) 'The effects of an ergonomic-educational course. Postural load, perceived physical exertion, and biomechanical errors in nursing', *International Archives of Occupational & Environmental Health* 71: 336–42.

Engkvist, I-L., Kjellberg, A., Wigaeus, H.E., Hagberg, M., Menckel, E. and Ekenvall, L. (2001) 'Back injuries among nursing personnel – identification of work conditions with cluster analysis', *Safety Science* 37: 1–18.

Entwistle, M., Horman, M., Lister, L. and Rimeur, G. (1996) 'Safe manual lifting of patients', *Journal of the Association for Quality in Healthcare* 3 (3): 118–24.

Essex Group of National Back Exchange (1996) *Paediatric Moving and Handling*: Report of workshops.

Evanoff, B.A., Bohr, P.C. and Wolf, L.D. (1999) 'Effects of a participatory ergonomics team among hospital orderlies', *American Journal of Industrial Medicine* 35 (4): 358–65.

Faculty of Occupational Medicine (2000) *Occupational Health Guidelines for the Management of Low Back Pain at Work: Evidence Review and Recommendations*, London: Faculty of Occupational Medicine, 27-8.

Fanello, S., Frampas-Chotard, V., Roquelaure, Y., Jousset, N., Delbos, V., Jarmy, J. and Penneau-Fontbonne, D. (1999) 'Evaluation of an educational low back pain prevention program for hospital employees', *Revue Du Rhumatisme* (Eng. edn) 66 (12): 711–16.

Fazel, E. (1998) 'The pain of moving', *Occupational Health* August: 22–3.

Feldstein, A., Valanis, B., Vollmer, W., Stevens, N. and Overton, C. (1993) 'The back injury prevention project pilot study. Assessing the effectiveness of back attack, an injury prevention program among nurses, aides, and orderlies', *Journal of Occupational Medicine* 35: 114–20.

Fenety, A. and Kumar, S. (1992) 'An ergonomic survey of a hospital physical therapy department', *International Journal of Industrial Ergonomics* 9: 161–70.

Foster, L. (1966) 'Manual handing training and changes in work practices', *Occupational Health* 48: 402–6.

Finsen, L., Christensen, H. and Bakke, M. (1998) 'Musculoskeletal disorders among dentists and variation in dental work', *Applied Ergonomics* 29: 119–25.

Fourie, J.A., Lief, E.M.P. and Dunne, T.T. (1992) 'Pillow positioning facilitates independent bridging for bedpan use in pelvic fractures', *South African Journal of Physiotherapy* 48 (3): 41–4.

Fragala, G. (1993) 'Injuries cut with lift use in ergonomics demonstration project', *Provider*, October: 39–40.

Fragala, G. and Santamaria, D. (1997) 'Heavy duties', *Health Facilities Management* 10 (5).

French, P., Lee Fung Wah, F., Sum Ping, L. and Wong Heung Yee, R. (1997) 'The prevalence and cause of occupational back pain in Hong Kong registered nurses', *Journal of Advanced Nursing* 26: 380–8.

Furber, S., Moore, H., Williamson, M. and Barry, J. (1997) 'Injuries to ambulance officers caused by patient handling tasks', *Journal of Occupational Health & Safety – Australia & New Zealand* 13 (3): 259–65.

Gabbett, J. (1998) 'A pilot study to investigate the lifting and sliding of patients up in bed', unpublished M.Sc. dissertation, University of Surrey.

Gagnon, M. and Lortie, M.A. (1987) 'Biomechanical approach to low-back problems in nursing aides', in Asfour, S. (ed.) *Trends in Ergonomics/Human Factors IV*, Holland: Elsevier Science Publishers B.V., 795–802.

Gagnon, M., Chehade, A., Kemp, F. and Lortie, M. (1987) 'Lumbo-sacral loads and selected muscle activity while turning patients in bed', *Ergonomics* 30 (7): 1013–32.

Gagnon, M., Roy, D. and Lortie, M. (1988a) 'The risks associated with changes of direction of the movement when handling patients: a biomechanical approach', *Ergonomics International 88: Proceedings of the 10th Congress of IEA*, Paris: The International Ergonomics Association, 123–5.

Gagnon, M., Roy, D., Lortie, M. and Roy, R. (1988b) 'Evolution of the execution parameters on a patient handling task', *Le Travail Humain* 51 (3): 193–210.

Gagnon, M., Sicard, C. and Sirois, J.P. (1986) 'Evaluation of forces on the lumbo-sacral joint and assessment of work and energy transfers in nursing aides lifting patients', *Ergonomics* 29 (3): 407–21.

Garb, J.R. and Dockery, C.A. (1995) 'Reducing employee back injuries in the perioperative setting', *AORN Journal* 61 (6): 1046–52.

Garg, A. and Owen, B. (1991) 'A biomechanical and ergonomic evaluation of patient transferring tasks', *Proceedings of 11th Congress of IEA*, Paris: The International Ergonomics Association, 1: 60–2.

Garg, A. and Owen, B. (1994) 'Prevention of back injuries in healthcare workers', *International Journal of Industrial Ergonomics* 14: 315–31.

Garg, A. and Owen, B. (1992) 'Reducing back stress in nursing personnel: an ergonomic intervention in a nursing home', *Ergonomics* 35 (11): 1353–75.

Garg, A., Owen, B. and Carlson, B. (1992) 'An ergonomic evaluation of nursing assistants' job in a nursing home', *Ergonomics* 35 (9): 979–95.

Garg, A., Owen, B., Beller, D. and Banaag, J.A., (1991a) 'Biomechanical and ergonomic evaluation of patient transferring tasks: bed to wheelchair and wheelchair to bed', *Ergonomics* 34 (3): 289–312.

Garg, A., Owen, B., Beller, D. and Banaag, J. (1991b) 'A biochemical and ergonomic evaluation of patient transferring tasks: wheelchair to shower chair and shower chair to wheelchair', *Ergonomics* 34 (4): 407–19.

Garrett, R.B. and Johnson Perry, A. (1996) 'A safer way to move patients', *Occupational Health and Safety*: 60–4.

Gingher, M.C., Karuza, J., Skulski, M.D. and Katz, P. (1996) 'Effectiveness of lift systems for long term care residents', *Physical and Occupational Therapy in Geriatrics* 14 (2): 1–11.

Goodridge, D. and Laurila, B. (1997) 'Minimizing transfer injuries', *The Canadian Nurse* 93 (7): 38–41.

Graham, J., Hurran, C. and MacKenzie, M. (2000) *Paediatric Manual Handling. Guidelines for Paediatric Physiotherapy*, Long Eaton: Association of Chartered Physiotherapists.

Gray, J., Cass, J., Harper, D.W. and O'Hara, P.A. (1996) 'A controlled evaluation of a lift and transfer educational program for nurses', *Geriatric Nursing* 17 (2): 81–5.

Green, C. (1996) 'Study of the moving and handling practices on two medical wards', *British Journal of Nursing* 5 (5): 303–11.

Grbich, C. (1999) *Qualitative Research in Health. An Introduction*, London: Sage Publications.

Griffiths, J. and McArthur, M. (1999) 'A qualitative study exploring the meaning of manual handing training in a working environment at risk of back injury', *Advancing Clinical Nursing* 3: 179–186.

Haigh, C. (1993) 'A study of micro-organism levels on nurses' footwear', *British Journal of Nursing* 2 (22): 1109–12.

Hamer, S. and Collinson, G. (1999) *Achieving Evidenced-based practice. A handbook for Practitioners*, Edinburgh: Ballière Tindall.

Hampton, S. (1998) 'Can electric beds aid pressure sore prevention in hospitals?' *British Journal of Nursing* 7 (17): 1010–17.

Harber, P., Pena, L., Hsu, P., Billet, E., Greer, D. and Kim, K. (1994) 'Personal history, training, and worksite as predictors of back pain of nurses', *American Journal of Industrial Medicine* 25: 519–26.

Hart, C. (1998) *Doing a literature review. Releasing the Social Science Research Imagination*, London: Sage Publications.

Head, M. and Levick, P. (1996) 'Patient handling: an ergonomic intervention', in *Proceedings of the 32nd Annual Ergonomics Society of Australia and the Safety Institute of Australia National Conference 1996, 'Enhancing Human Performance'*, 22–5 September 1996, Australia: Canberra.

Health Services Advisory Committee (1998) *Manual Handling in the Health Services*, Health and Safety Commission, London: HMSO.

Hellsing, A.L., Linson, S.J., Andershed, B., Bergman, C. and Liew, M. (1993) 'Ergonomic education for nursing students', *International Journal of Nursing Studies* 30: 499–510.

Hignett, S. (1996a) 'Manual handling risks in midwifery: identification of risk factors', *British Journal of Midwifery* 4 (11): 590–6.

Hignett, S. (1996b) 'Work-related back pain in nurses', *Journal of Advanced Nursing* 23: 1238–46.

Hignett, S. (1998) 'Ergonomic evaluation of electric mobile hoists', *British Journal of Occupational Therapy* 61 (11): 509–16.

Hignett, S. (1999) 'East Midlands Group: ergonomic produce evaluation sliding sheets', *The Column* 11 (1): 20–4.

Hignett, S. (2001a) 'Manual handling risk assessments in occupational therapy', *British Journal of Occupational Therapy* 64 (2): 81–6.

Hignett, S. (2001b) 'Embedding ergonomics in hospital culture: top-down and bottom-up strategies', *Applied Ergonomics* 32: 61–9.

Hignett, S. and Richardson, B. (1995) 'Manual handling human loads in a hospital: an exploratory study to identify nurses' perceptions', *Applied Ergonomics* 26 (3): 221–6.

Holliday, P.J., Fernie, G.R. and Plowman, S. (1994) 'The impact of new lifting technology in long term care', *AAOHN Journal* 42 (12): 582–9.

Hui, L., Ng, G.Y.F., Yeung, S.S.M. and Hui-Chan, C.W.Y. (2001) 'Evaluation of physiological work demands and low back neuromuscular fatigue on nurses working in geriatric wards', *Applied Ergonomics* 32: 479–83.

Human Services/Victorian Work cover Authority (1999) *Manual Handling: Reducing the Risk, Reducing Injuries*, Australia: Human Services/Victorian Work cover Authority.

Jackson, J. and Liles, C. (1994) 'Working postures and physiotherapy students', *Physiotherapy* 80 (7): 432–6.

Johnston, M. 'Handle with care', (1987) *Senior Nurse* 6 (5): 20–2.

Kato, M., Muzima, M. and Nishiguchi, H. (2000) 'Application of industrial method to care work', *Proceedings of the IEA2000/HFES 2000 Congress*, The Human Factors and Ergonomics Society, California: Santa Monica, 4: 268.

Khalil, T.M., Asfour, S.S., Marchette, B. and Omachonu, V. (1987) 'Lower back injuries in nursing: a biomechanical analysis and intervention strategy' in Asfour, S.S. (ed.) *Trends in Ergonomics/Human Factors IV*, Holland: Elsevier Science Publishers B.V., 811–21.

Kilbom, A., Ljungberg, A.S. and Hägg, G. (1985) 'Lifting and carrying in geriatric care. A comparison between differences in workspace layout, work organisation and use of modern equipment', in Brown I. *et al.* (eds) *Ergonomics International* 85: 550–3.

King, L. (1994) 'Safe handling of hip replacement patients', *Nursing Standard* 8 (47): 31–5.

Kitson, J. (2000) 'Mind your back: variable height cots', *Paediatric Nursing* 12 (4): 26–7.

Knapik, J.J., Harper, W., Crowell, H.P., Leiter, K. and Mull, B. (2000) 'Standard and alternative methods of stretcher carriage: performance, human factors, and cardio-respiratory responses', *Ergonomics* 43 (5): 639–52.

Knibbe, J.J. and Friele, R.D. (1999) 'The use of logs to assess exposure to manual handling of patients, illustrated in an intervention study in home care nursing', *International Journal of Industrial Ergonomics* 24: 445–54.

Knibbe, J.J. and Friele, R.D. (1996) 'Prevalence of back pain and characteristics of the physical workload of community nurses', *Ergonomics* 39 (2): 186–98.

Knibbe, N., and Knibbe, J.J. (1995) 'Postural load of nurses during bathing and showering of patients', Internal Report, *Locomotion Health Consultancy*, The Netherlands.

Kothiyal, K. and Yuen, T.W. (2000) 'Manual handling in nursing jobs: an ergonomic study of a patient transferring aid', *Proceedings of the IEA2000/HFES 2000 Congress*, The Human Factors and Ergonomics Society, California: Santa Monica, 5: 610.

Laflin, K. and Aja, D. (1995) 'Health care concerns related to lifting: an inside look at intervention strategies', *American Journal of Occupational Therapy* 49: 63–72.

Lagerström, M. and Hagberg, M. (1997) 'Evaluation of a three year education and training program for nursing personnel at a Swedish Hospital', *AAOHN Journal* 45 (2): 83–92.

Lavender, S.A., Conrad, K.M., Reichelt, P.A., Johnson, P.W. and Meyer, F.T. (2000a). 'Biomechanical analyses of paramedics simulating frequently performed strenuous work tasks', *Applied Ergonomics* 31: 167–77.

Lavender, S.A., Conrad, K.M., Reichelt, P.A., Meyer, F.T. and Johnson, P.W. (2000b) 'Postural analysis of paramedics simulating frequently performed strenuous work tasks', *Applied Ergonomics*. 31 (1): 45–57.

Lavender, S.A., Thomas, J.S., Chang, D. and Andersson, G.B.J. (1995) 'Effect of lifting belts, foot movement, and lift asymmetry on trunk motions', *Human Factors* 37 (4): 844–53.

Le Bon, C. and Forrester, C. (1997) 'An ergonomic evaluation of a patient handling device: the elevate and transfer vehicle', *Applied Ergonomics* 28 (5/6): 365–74.

Lee, Y.H. and Chiou, W.K. (1994) 'Risk factors for low back pain, and patient-handling capacity of nursing personnel', *Journal of Safety Research* 25 (3): 135–45.

Lindbeck, L. and Engkvist, I.L. (1993) 'Biomechanical analysis of two patient handling tasks', *International Journal of Industrial Ergonomics* 12: 117–25.

Ljungberg, A.S., Kilborn, A. and Hägg, G. (1989) 'Occupational lifting by nursing aides and warehouse workers', *Ergonomics* 32 (1): 59–78.

Lloyd, P., Tarling, C., Troup, J.D.G. and Wright, B. (1987) *The Handling of Patients. A guide for Nurses* (2nd edn) Back Pain Association/Royal College of Nursing.

Lloyd, P., Fletcher, B., Holmes, D., Tarling, C. and Tracy, M. (1998, revised) *The Guide to the Handling of Patients* (4th edn) National Back Pain Association/Royal College of Nursing.

Love, C. (1986) 'Do you roll or lift?' *Nursing Times* 82 (29): 44–6.

Love, C. (1994) 'Rolling or lifting following hip replacement', *Professional Nurse* April: 456–64.

Love, C. (1996a) 'Injury caused by lifting: a study of the nurse's viewpoint', *Nursing Standard*. 10 (46): 34–9.

Love, C. (1996b) 'Ergonomic considerations when choosing a hoist and slings', *British Journal of Therapy and Rehabilitation* 3 (4): 189–98.

Luntley, J. and Pearce, J. (1995) 'Lifting and handling of patients by anaesthetists', *Anaesthesia* 50: 729–32.

Lusted, M.J., Carrasco, C.L., Mandryk, J.A. and Healey, S. (1996) 'Self reported symptoms in the neck and upper limbs in nurses', *Applied Ergonomics* 27 (6): 381–7.

Lynch, R.M. and Freund, A. (2000) 'Short-term efficacy of back injury intervention project for patient care providers at one hospital', AIHAJ: *Journal for the Science of Occupational & Environmental Health & Safety* 61: 290–4.

MacKenzie, M., Richardson, B., Kidd, R. and Tracy, M. (1997) 'A novel limb-support system to reduce postural load in theatres', *British Journal of Theatre Nursing* 6 (10): 28–30.

Manual Handling (MHOR) (1992) *Manual Handling Operations Regulations 1992 Guidance for Regulations*, L23 (2nd edn, 1998) London: HSE Books.

Marras, W.S., Davis, K.G., Kirking, B.C. and Bertsche, P.K. (1999) 'A comprehensive analysis of low-back disorder risk and spinal loading during the transferring and repositioning of patients using different techniques', *Ergonomics* 42 (7): 904–26.

Massad, R., Gambin, C. and Duval. L. (2000) 'The contribution of ergonomics to the prevention of musculoskeletal lesions among ambulance technicians', *Proceedings of the IEA2000/HFES 2000 Congress,* The Human Factors and Ergonomics Society, California: Santa Monica, 4: 201–4.

McGill, S.M., Potvin, J. and Norman, R.W. (1990) 'Estimating low back demands in ambulance attendants using a hybrid anatomical model', *Proceedings of the 23rd conference of the Human Factors Association of Canada, Ottawa, Canada,* Ontario: The Association, Mississauga, 191–5.

McGuire, T. and Dewar, J. (1995) 'An assessment of moving and handling practices among Scottish nurses', *Nursing Standard* 9 (40): 35–9.

McGuire, T., Moody, J., Hanson, M., and Tigar, F. (1996a) 'A study into clients' attitudes towards mechanical aids', *Nursing Standard* 11 (5): 35–8.

McGuire, T., Moody, J. and Hanson, M. (1996b) 'An evaluation of mechanical aids used within the NHS', *Nursing Standard* 11 (6): 33–8.

McGuire, T., Moody, J. and Hanson, M. (1997) 'Managers' attitudes towards mechanical aids', *Nursing Standard* 11 (31): 33–8.

McKellar, N.B. and Shaw, H. (1986) 'Back breaking work (lifting patients in the operating theatre)', *NATNEWS* 23: 14–16.

MDA (1994) *Slings to Accompany Mobile Domestic Hoists,* Norwich: HMSO: A10.

MDA (1996) *Moving and Transferring Equipment,* Norwich: HMSO: A19.

MDA (1997) *Handling Equipment for Moving Dependent People in Bed,* Norwich: HMSO: A23.

Menckel, E., Hagberg, M., Engkvist, I.L. and Wigaeus-Hjelm, E. (1997) 'The prevention of back injuries in Swedish health care – a comparison between two models for action-oriented feedback', *Applied Ergonomics* 28 (1): 1–7.

Menoni, O., Battevi, N., Colombini, D., Ricci, D., Occhipinti, E. and Zecchi, G. (1999) 'Assessment of risk due to manual lifting of patients', *Giornale Italiano di Medicina del Lavoro* 90 (2): 191–200.

Meyer, E. (1995) 'Patient lifter in a practical test. A spine-saving aid or bulk in the storage room?' *Pflege Aktuell* 49 (9): 597–600.

Miller, M. and Johnston, C. (1992) 'Moving and handling skills for carers', *TES Crossroads,* 1–28.

Mital, A. and Shrey, D.E., (1996) 'Back problems in health professionals: extent of the problem and an integrated approach for its management', *Critical Reviews in Physical and Rehabilitation Medicine* 8 (3): 201–19.

Mitchell, J, Jones, J., McNair, B. and McClenahan, J.W. (1998) *Better Beds for Health Care: Report of the King's Fund Centenary Bed Project,* London: King's Fund.

Monaghan, H., Robinson, L. and Steele, Y. (1998) 'Implementing a no lift policy', *Nursing Standard* 12 (50): 35–7.

Moody, J., McGuire, T., Hanson, M. and Tigar, F. (1996) 'A study of nurses' attitudes towards mechanical aids', *Nursing Standard* 11 (4): 37–42.

Mulligan, K.S. and Webb, L.Z. (1988) 'Developing an evacuation procedure for a nursery complex', *Neonatal Network* 6: 47–52.

Murphy, E., Dingwall, R., Greatbatch, D., Parker, S. and Watson, P. (1998) 'Qualitative research methods in health technology assessment: a review of the literature', *Health Technol Assessment* 2, 16. http://www.soton.ac.uk/~hts.

Nestor, D. (1988) 'Hospital bed design and operation – effect on incidence of low back injuries among nursing personnel', in Aghazadeh, F. (ed.) *Trends in Ergonomics/ Human Factors V,* Holland: Elsevier Science Publishers B.V., 729–40.

Newman, S. and Callaghan, C. (1993) 'Work-related back pain', *Occupational Health* 45: 201–5.

Ng, C., Phongsathorn, V. and Mitchell, S. (1997) 'Doctors should be trained in lifting patients', *British Medical Journal* 315: 551.

NIOSH (1981) *Work Practices Guide for Manual Lifting,* DHSS (NIOSH), Ohio: Cincinatti, 81:122.

Norton, L. (2000) 'An ergonomic evaluation into fabric slings used during the hoisting of patients', unpublished M.Sc. dissertation, University of Nottingham.

Nussbaum, M.A. and Torres, N. (2001) 'Effects of training in modifying working methods during common patient-handling activities', *International Journal of Industrial Ergonomics* 27: 33–41.

Nyran, P.I. (1991) 'Cost effectiveness of core-group training', in Karwowski, W. and Yates, J. W. (eds) *Advances in Industrial Ergonomics and Safety III,* London: Taylor & Francis, 778–82.

Oddy, R. (1993) 'Legislation in action: must we lift?' *Physiotherapy* 79 (12): 827–30.

Olsson, G. and Brandt, A. (1992) 'An investigation of the use of ceiling mounted hoists for disabled people', Demark: Danish centre for technical aids for rehabilitation and education.

Overd, A. (1992) 'Should we lift or should we roll? Nursing practice following prosthetic hip surgery', *Professional Nurse* 7: 311–19.

Owen, B. (1987) 'The need for application of ergonomic principles in nursing', in Asfour, S. (ed.) *Trends in Ergonomics/Human Factors IV,* Holland: Elsevier Science Publishers B.V., 831–8.

Owen, B.D. (1988) 'Patient handling devices: an ergonomic approach to lifting patients', in Aghazadeh, F. (ed.) *Trends in Ergonomics/Human Factors V,* Holland: Elsevier Science Publishers B.V., 721–8.

Owen, B. (1999) 'Decreasing the back injury problem in nursing personnel', *Surgical Services Management* 5 (7): 15–21.

Owen, B. and Hasler-Hanson, C.R. (1999) 'A study comparing three methods of repositioning "patients" up in bed', *Journal of Healthcare Safety Compliance and Infection Control* 3 (8): 362–7.

Owen, B., Garg, A. and Jensen, R.C. (1992) 'Four methods for identification of most back-stressing tasks performed by nursing assistants in nursing homes', *International Journal of Industrial Ergonomics* 9: 213–20.

Owen, B.D. and Fragala, G. (1999) 'Reducing perceived physical stress while transferring residents: an ergonomic approach', *AAOHN Journal* 47: 316–23.

Owen, B. and Garg, A. (1989) 'Patient handling tasks perceived to be most stressful by nursing assistants', in Mital, A. (ed.) *Advances in Industrial Ergonomics and Safety*, London: Taylor & Francis, 775–81.

Owen, B.D. and Garg, A. (1994) 'Reducing back stress through an ergonomic approach: weighing a patient', *International Journal of Nursing Studies* 31: 511–19.

Owen, B.D., Welden, N. and Kane, J. (1999) 'What are we teaching about lifting and transferring patients?', *Research in Nursing and Health* 22 (3): 3–13.

Oxford Region, National Back Exchange (1999) *Generic Safe Systems of Work for Patient Handling and Inanimate Load Management*, Oxford Region: National Back Exchange.

Pain, H., Jackson, S., McLellan, D.L. and Gore, S. (1999) 'User evaluation of handling equipment for moving dependent people in bed', *Technology & Disability* 11: 13–19.

Pan, C-C. and Freivalos, A. (2000) 'Ergonomic evaluation of a new patient handling device', *Proceedings of the IEA2000/HFES 2000 Congress*, The Human Factors and Ergonomics Society, California: Santa Monica, 4: 274.

Panciera, D., Menoni, O. and Ricci, M. (2000) 'Hoists; selection criteria and standards', *Proceedings of the IEA2000/HFES 2000 Congress*, The Human Factors and Ergonomics Society, California: Santa Monica, 5: 797–800.

Paternoster, D., Salis, M. and Gisser, G.V. (1999) 'An experience in training of hospital staff with tasks involving manual load lifting in Bressanone Hospital: content and checking of efficacy', *Giornale Italiano di Medicina del Lavoro* 90 (2): 381–92.

Peers, M.L. (1998) 'Prevention of nursing strain injuries in the long term care setting: the Fairview Lodge experience', *Perspectives* 22 (1): 23–4.

Petzäll J. (1996) 'Traversing step obstacles with manual wheelchairs', *Applied Ergonomics* 27 (5): 327–41.

Pohjonen, T., Punakallio, A. and Louhevaara, V. (1998) 'Participatory ergonomics for reducing load and strain in home care work', *International Journal of Industrial Ergonomics* 21: 345–52.

Proteau, R.A. (2000) 'Ergonomics in home care', *Proceedings of the IEA2000/HFES 2000 Congress*, The Human Factors and Ergonomics Society, California: Santa Monica, 4: 275.

Quintana, R. and Alonso, J. (1997) 'An ergonomic patient-handling methodology', *Proceedings of the Silicon Valley Ergonomics Conference & Exposition*, California: San Jose University, 67–74.

Raistrick, A. (1981) 'Nurses with back pain – can the problem be prevented?' *Nursing Times*, May 14: 853–6.

Revie, M. (2000) 'Manual handling of the deceased in the funeral industry', *The Column*, August: 17–20.

Robertson, H. (2000) 'The transfer slide sheet. A useful device to reduce nursing lifting demands', *Geriaction* 15 (2): 13–18.

Robertson, L.D., Changsut, R., Ramos, L.S. and Jones, D.W. (1993) 'Influence of job and personal risk factors on safety limits for kinesiotherapists performing a stressful clinical lifting task', *Clinical Kinesiology* 47 (1): 7–16.

Rodgers, S. (1985a) 'Shouldering the load', *Nursing Times*, January 16: 24–6.

Rodgers, S. (1985b) 'Positive lifting', *Nursing Times*, January 23: 43–5.

Roth, P.T., Ciecka, J., Wood, E.C. and Taylor, R. (1993) 'Evaluation of a unique mechanical client lift. Efficiency and perspectives of nursing staff', *AAOHN Journal* 41 (5): 229–34.

Royal College of Midwives (1997) *Handle with Care. A Midwife's Guide to Preventing Back Injury*, London: Royal College of Midwives.

Ruszala, S. (2001) 'An evaluation of equipment to assist patient sit-to-stand activities in physiotherapy', unpublished M.Sc. dissertation, University of Wales: School of Health Care Studies.

Santoro, M. (1994) 'Lifting teams can help hospitals eliminate costly back injuries to nurses', *Hospital Employee Health* 13 (7): 81–7.

Schibye, B. and Skotte, J. (2000) 'The mechanical loads on the low back during different patient handling tasks', *Proceedings of the IEA2000/HFES 2000 Congress*, The Human Factors and Ergonomics Society, California: Santa Monica, 5: 785–8.

Scholey, M. (1982) 'The shoulder lift', *Nursing Times*, March 24: 506–7.

Scholey, M. (1983) 'Back stress; the effects of training nurses to lift patients in a clinical situation', *International Journal of Nursing Studies* 20: 1–13.

Scopa, M. (1993) Comparison of classroom instruction and independent study in body mechanics', *The Journal of Continuing Education in Nursing* 24 (4): 170–3.

Scott, A. (1995) 'Improving patient moving and handling skills', *Professional Nurse* 109 (11): 105–6.

Seale, C. (1999) *The Quality of Qualitative Research*, London: Sage Publications.

Shrout, P.E. and Fleiss, J.L. (1979) 'Intraclass correlations: uses in assessing rater reliability', *Psychological Bulletin* 86: 420–8.

Skarplik, C. (1988) 'Patient handling in the community', *Nursing* 3 (30): 13–16.

Smedley, J., Egger, P., Cooper, C. and Coggon, D. (1995) 'Manual handling activities and risk of low back pain in nurses', *Occupational & Environmental Medicine* 52: 160–3.

South London and Kent Group, National Back Exchange (1998) *Manual Handling Procedures*, South London and Kent Group: National Back Exchange.

Sparkes, V. (2000) 'Physiotherapy for stroke rehabilitation: a need for evidence based handling techniques', *Physiotherapy* 86 (7): 348–56.

St Vincent, M., Tellier, C. and Lortie, M. (1989) 'Training in handling an evaluative study', *Ergonomics* 32 (2): 191–210.

Stevenson, M.G. (1995) 'Mechanics of lifting patients on ambulance stretchers', *Proceedings of the Ergonomics Society of Australia*, Glenelg, Adelaide, 135–42.

Stubbs, D.A. and Osborne, C. (1979) 'How to save your back. A comparison between the nursing profession and the construction industry', *Nursing*, 3: 116–24.

Stubbs, D.A., Buckle, P., Hudson, M.P. and Rivers, P.M. (1983) 'Back pain in the nursing profession – II. The effectiveness of training', *Ergonomics* 26 (8): 767–79.

Switzer, S. and Porter J.M. (1993) 'The lifting behaviour of nurses – in their own words', in Darby, F. and Turner, P. (eds) *Proc. 7th Conf. NZ Ergonomics Soc. 2–3 August 1996*, Wellington: New Zealand Ergonomics Society, 33–43.

Takala, E.P. and Kukkonen, R. (1987) 'The handling of patients on geriatric wards', *Applied Ergonomics* 18 (1): 17–22.

The Disability Information Trust (1996) *Hoists, Lifts and Transfers*, The Disability Information Trust, Oxford: Nuffield Orthopaedic Centre.

The Resuscitation Council (2001) *Guidance for Safer Handling During Resuscitation in Hospital*, London: The Resuscitation Council.

Thompson, E. (2000) 'Safer birthing positions. A choice for mother and midwife', *The Column* 12 (2): 17–22.

Torma-Krajewski, J. (1987) 'Analysis of lifting tasks in the health care industry', in

Occupational Hazards to Health Care Workers, American Conference of Governmental Industrial Hygienists, 51–68.

Torri, P., Liboni, D., Milan, F. and Piccoli, R. (1999) 'An experience in management of risk due to manual lifting of patients in hospitals in the Veneto Region', *Giornale Italiano di Medicina del Lavoro* 90 (2): 362–80.

Tracy, M. (1996) 'Campaign for safer patient handling', *Occupational Health* 48: 50–2.

Tracy, M. (1997) 'An ergonomic evaluation of slide sheets', *The Column:* 21–6.

Tracz, S. and Rose, I. (1982) 'Beating low back pain', *Dimensions in Health Service* 59: 20–3.

Trevelyan, F.C. (2001) 'The implementation and evaluation of an ergonomics intervention in a health care setting', Unpublished Ph.D. thesis, Robens Centre for Health Ergonomics, European Institute for Health and Medical Sciences, University of Surrey.

Troup, D., Lloyd, P., Osborne, C. and Tarling, C. (1981) *The Handling of Patients. A Guide for Nurse Managers,* Back Pain Association/Royal College of Nursing.

Troup, J.D. and Rauhala, H.H. (1987) 'Ergonomics and training', *International Journal of Nursing Studies* 24 (4): 325–30.

Tuffnell, C. (1989) 'Lightening the lifting load through education and quality assurance monitoring', *Australian Clinical Review* 9: 123–6.

Ukoumunne, O.C., Gulliford, M.C., Chinn, S., Sterne, J.A.C. and Burney, P.G.J. (1999) 'Methods for evaluating area-wide and organisation-based interventions in health and health-care: a systematic review, *Health Technol Assess* 3 (5).

Ulin, S., Chaffin, D.B., Patellos, C. and Blitz, S. (1997) 'A biomechanical analysis of methods used for transferring totally dependent patients', *Scientific Nursing* 14 (1): 19–27.

Varcin-Coad, L. and Barrett, R. (1998) 'Repositioning a slumped person in a wheelchair. A biomechanical analysis of three transfer techniques', *AAOHN Journal* 46 (11): 530–6.

Venning, P.J. (1988) 'Back injury prevention. Instructional design features for program planning', *AAOHN Journal* 36 (8): 336–41.

Videman, T., Rauhala, H., Asp, S., Lindström, K., Cedercreutz, G., Kämppi, M., Tola, S. and Troup, J.D.G. (1989) 'Patient-handling skill, back injuries, and back pain: an intervention study in nursing', *Occupational Health* 41: 148–56.

Wachs, J.E. and Parker, J.E. (1987) 'Registered nurses' lifting behaviour in the hospital setting', in Asfour, S. (ed.) *Trends in Ergonomics/Human Factors* IV, Holland: Elsevier Science, Publishers B.V., 883–90.

Waldenström, U. and Gottvall, K. (1991) 'A randomised trial of birthing stool of conventional semirecumbent position for second-stage labor', *Birth* 18 (1): 5–10.

Whalley-Hammell, K., Carpenter, C. and Dyck I. (2000) *Using Qualitative Research. A Practical Introduction for Occupational and Physical Therapists,* Edinburgh: Churchill Livingstone.

Winkelmolen, G.H.M., Landeweerd, J. and Drost, M.R. (1994) 'An evaluation of patient lifting techniques', *Ergonomics* 37 (5): 921–32.

Wood, D.J. (1987) 'Design and evaluation of a back injury prevention program within a geriatric hospital', *Spine* 12 (2): 77–82.

Wood, J., Raudsepp, T., Miller, L. and Dazey, E. (2000) 'Improving resident transfers', *Nursing: Long Term Management,* June: 68–76.

Wright, A., Smith, L.A. and Landers, J. (1991) 'Design and evaluation of an ergonomic patient lifting device', *Advances in Industrial Ergonomics & Safety,* London: Taylor & Francis, 3: 293–9.

Wright, B. (1981a) 'Lifting and moving patients: 1. an investigation and commentary', *Nursing Times,* November 11: 1962–5.

Wright, B. (1981b) 'Lifting and moving patients: 2. training and management', *Nursing Times*, November 18: 2025–8.

Zelenka, J.P., Floren, A.E. and Jordan, J.J. (1996) 'Minimal forces to move patients', *American Journal of Occupational Therapy* 50 (5): 354–61.

Zhuang, Z., Stobbe, T.J., Collins, J.W., Hsiao, H., and Hobbs, G.R. (2000) 'Psycho-physical assessment of assistive devices for transferring patients/residents', *Applied Ergonomics* 31: 35–44.

Zhuang, Z., Stobbe, T.J., Hsiao, H., Collins, J.W. and Hobbs, G.R. (1999) 'Bio-mechanical evaluation of assistive devices for transferring residents', *Applied Ergonomics* 30: 285–94.

GLOSSARY

This glossary has been compiled assuming some knowledge of health care. The terminology relates to:

- measurement tools; and
- abbreviations.

Where terms are both measurement tools and abbreviations they are listed under measurement tools. Some terms vary throughout the text depending on factors such as country of origin. We have kept to the terminology used in the original paper as far as possible. This means that there are a number of different terms with the same meaning such as patient/client or hoist/lifter.

The definitions of the study types can be found in Chapter 2. Definitions of equipment are not included due to the wide range of terminology; however, any detail from the original paper has been included in the abstract.

If any further information or explanation is required please consult the original paper.

Measurement tools

AL	Action Limit (NIOSH)
ARB5	A biomechanical model
BPDS	Body Part Discomfort Scale. A paper-and-pen self-reporting tool, collecting information about aches and pains and their location
Biomechanical modelling	Various methods of measuring changes in body posture
Cinematography	Use of video (moving pictures) for data collection
EMG	Electromyography. The measurement of electrical activity in a muscle
Force platform	A measurement device for measuring forces exerted by body parts
GHQ	General Health Questionnaire
IAP	Intra-abdominal pressure calculation that equates with force acting on the lumbar spine
Likert scale	A scale used to quantify responses in a questionnaire
LMM	Lumbar Motion Monitor. An electronic goniometer for measuring the range of motion in the spine
MAPO	Index of exposure to identify prevention and improve measures

MPL	Maximal Permissible Limit (NIOSH)
NIOSH	National Institute of Occupational Safety and Health
	Terms used by NIOSH to define weight limits include:
Nordic questionnaire	A questionnaire to collect data on musculoskeletal discomfort
NUD*IST	Non-numerical Unstructured Data Indexing Searching and Theorising: a qualitative data-management computer programme
OWAS	Ovako Working posture Analysis System: a paper-and-pen postural analysis tool
PEO	Portable Ergonomic Observation: a computerised postural analysis tool
REBA	Rapid Entire Body Assessment: a paper-and-pen postural analysis tool
RPE (Borg scale)	Rated Perceived Exertion: a validated self-reported scale of perceived exertion
WAI	Work Ability Index: assessment tool collecting data on the worker's own assessment of his or her work ability
WATBAK	A postural analysis tool
WHQ	Work and Health Questionnaire

Abbreviations

2D	2-dimensional: movement only in a sagittal plane
3D	3-dimensional: movement in a sagittal or coronal plane, including twisting and rotation
CPR	Cardiopulmonary resuscitation
ILO	International Labour Office
L4/5	4th and 5th lumbar vertebrae
LBP	Low-Back Pain
MHOR	Manual Handling Operations Regulations (UK)
PO	Professional Opinion
PR	Practitioner Rating (Hignett's convincing scale, see Appendix 2 on page 188)
QR	Quality Rating (see Appendix 2 on page 188)
VAS	Visual Analogue Scale

EXAMPLE OF MEDLINE SEARCH FROM 1960–2001

String Search

1	(manual adj4 handl$).tw.
2	(patient adj4 handl$).tw.
3	(patient adj4 lift$).tw.
4	(patient adj4 mov$).tw.
5	(patient adj4 transfer$).tw.
6	(patient adj4 carr$).tw.
7	1 or 2 or 3 or 4 or 5 or 6
8	(hospital bed$ adj4 handl$).tw.
9	(hospital bed$ adj4 lift$).tw.
10	(hospital bed$ adj4 mov$).tw.
11	(hospital bed$ adj4 transfer$).tw.
12	(theatre$ adj4 handl$).tw.
13	(theatre$ adj4 lift$).tw.
14	(theatre$ adj4 mov$).tw.
15	(theatre$ adj4 transfer$).tw.
16	(wheelchair$ adj4 handl$).tw.
17	(wheelchair$ adj4 lift$).tw.
18	(theatre$ adj4 mov$).tw.
19	(theatre$ adj4 transfer$).tw.
20	lifting belt$.tw
21	(toilet$ adj4 handl$).tw.
22	(toilet$ adj4 lift$).tw.
23	(toilet$ adj4 mov$).tw.
24	(toilet$ adj4 transfer$).tw.
25	(bath$ adj4 handl$).tw.
26	(bath$ adj4 lift$).tw.
27	(bath$ adj4 mov$).tw.
28	(bath$ adj4 transfer$).tw.
29	(helicopter$ adj4 handl$).tw.
30	(helicopter$ adj4 lift$).tw.
31	(helicopter$ adj4 mov$).tw.
32	(helicopter$ adj4 transfer$).tw.
33	(stretcher$ adj4 handl$).tw.
34	(stretcher$ adj4 lift$).tw.
35	(stretcher$ adj4 mov$).tw.
36	(stretcher$ adj4 transfer$).tw.

37	(stretcher$ adj4 carr$).tw.
38	8 or 10 or 11 or 12 or 13 or 14 or 15 or 16 or 17 or 18 or 19 or 20 or 21 or 22 or 23 or 24 or 25 or 26 or 27 or 28 or 29 or 30 or 31 or 32 or 33 or 34 or 35 or 36 or 37
39	exp health personnel/
40	exp nursing/
41	nursing.tw.
42	nurse.tw.
43	nurses.tw.
44	equipment design/or 'facility design and construction'/or 'hospital design and construction'/or 'interior design and furnishings'/
45	'equipment and supplies'/or 'equipment and supplies, hospital'/or protective devices/or self-help devices/or surgical equipment/
46	exp human engineering/
47	exp man-machine systems/
48	exp task performance analysis/
49	exp biomechanics/
50	exp lifting/
51	lift$.tw.
52	hoist$.tw.
53	ergonomic$.tw.
54	human factors.tw.
55	exp risk assessment/
56	accidents/or accident prevention/or accidents, occupational/
57	exp 'wounds and injuries'/
58	arm injuries/or back injuries/or contusions/or hand injuries/or leg injuries/or neck injuries/or soft tissue injuries/or spinal injuries/or 'sprains and strains'/or tendon injuries/or thoracic injuries/
59	exp back pain/
60	exp transportation of patients/
61	39 or 40 or 41 or 42 or 43
62	7 or 38 or 44 or 45 or 46 or 47 or 48 or 49 or 50 or 51 or 52 or 53 or 54 or 55 or 60
63	56 or 57 or 58 or 59
64	61 and 62 and 63

DATA APPRAISAL/ EXTRACTION FORMS

The questions in this checklist (Sections A, B, C and D) have been reproduced with the kind permission of Professor Nick Black, Professor of Health Services Research, London School of Hygiene and Tropical Medicine, University of London and BMJ Publishing Group.

The questions are taken from:
Downs, S.H. and Black, N. (1998) 'The feasibility of creating a check list for the assessment of the methodological quality both of randomised and non-randomised studies of health care interventions', *J Epidemiol Community Health* 52: 377–84.

CRITICAL APPRAISAL AND DATA EXTRACTION FORM

(should take from 10–45 minutes per paper)

Reviewer identification (please write your name in this box)

Paper identification number:
Author(s):
Year:
Title:

Is the paper about:

A patient-handling task?   ☐
Patient-handling equipment?   ☐
An intervention related to patient handling (including training and   ☐
ergonomic changes)?

Exclude paper for the following reasons:

Please list tasks/equipment/intervention strategy:

1

2

3

4

5

6

Type of study classification

Type of study?		Which section?	
Trial with an intervention/RCT/experimental	☐	Section A	☐
Trial without an intervention/ non-RCT/quasi-experimental	☐		
Controlled observational study		Section B	☐
Cohort study	☐		
Case–control study	☐		
Observational study without controls		Section C	☐
Cross-sectional study	☐		
Survey	☐		
Case series	☐	Section D	☐
Qualitative study	☐	Section E	☐
Professional opinion	☐	Section F	☐

What is/are the hypothesis/aim/ objective(s)? (There may be more than one reported in the paper) **Section A, B, C, D, E**	
Which population group was used? (e.g. nurses, patients, carers?) **Section A, B, C, D, E**	
What are the interventions? Section A	
What are the main outcome measures? (There may be more than one, list all the measures used) **Section A, B, C, D**	
What are the main findings of the study? Section A, B, C, D, E	

Section A

1A	
2A	
3A	
4A	
5A	
6A	
7A	
8A	
9A	
10A	
11A	
12A	
13A	
14A	
15A	
16A	
17A	
18A	
19A	
20A	
21A	
22A	
23A	
24A	
25A	
26A	
Score (27)	

Section B

1B	
2B	
3B	
4B	
5B	
6B	
7B	
8B	
9B	
10B	
11B	
12B	
13B	
15B	
16B	
17B	
18B	
19B	
20B	
21B	
22B	
25B	
26B	
Score (24)	

Section C

1C	
2C	
2Ci	
3C	
5C	
6C	
7C	
8C	
9C	
10C	
11C	
12C	
13C	
15C	
16C	
18C	
20C	
21C	
22C	
25C	
26C	
Score (22)	

Section D

1D	
3D	
6D	
9D	
10D	
11D	
12D	
13D	
18D	
20D	
21D	
22D	
26D	
Score	

Section E

27	
28	
29	
30	
31	
32	
33	
34	
35	
36	
37	
38	
39	
Score	

Section F
Questions about professional opinion or consensus

Was 'expert' defined? How and by whom?	

Was this a consensus of opinions? What processes were used for the final decision-making agreement?	

Were any processes of external review undertaken? (e.g. external examiner for a thesis or dissertation) *Comments*	Yes No Unable to determine	☐ ☐ ☐
Who funded the process?	Unable to determine	☐

Section G
Your summary of this paper

1 Summarise the *relevant* research/evaluation/assessment question:

2 Summarise the conclusion:

3 Hignett's 'convincing' scale
   How convinced are you, as a practitioner, by the relevant findings or recommendations from this paper?

   Very convinced, will definitely use in my practice/teaching ☐
   Fairly convinced, might use in my practice/teaching ☐
   Borderline, there might be something in this, but I need to know more ☐
   Not convinced. But I don't think this is complete rubbish ☐
   Complete rubbish! ☐

Please explain why you have given the above grade: e.g. methodological quality, reality check (for lab. study), personal experience or whatever.

Section A
Experimental or quasi-experimental

1A Is the hypothesis/aim/objective of the study clearly described?	Yes	☐ 1
	No	☐ 0
2A Are the main outcomes to be measured clearly described in the Introduction or Methods section?	Yes	☐ 1
	No	☐ 0
If the main outcomes are first mentioned in the Results section, the question should be answered 'no'.		
3A Sampling: Are the characteristics of the subjects included in the study clearly described?	Yes	☐ 1
	No	☐ 0
Inclusion and/or exclusion criteria should be given.		
4A Are the interventions of interest clearly described?	Yes	☐ 1
Equipment or changes in technique that are to be compared should be clearly described.	No	☐ 0
5A Are the distributions of the principal confounders in each group of subjects to be compared clearly described?	Yes	☐ 2
	Partially	☐ 1
(Confounding variable = an unforeseen and unaccounted for variable that jeopardises reliability and validity of an experiment outcome.)	No	☐ 0
6A Are the main findings of the study clearly described?	Yes	☐ 1
Simple outcome data should be reported for all major findings so that the reader can check the major analyses and conclusions (see Question 18 for statistical tests).	No	☐ 0
7A Does the study provide estimates of the random variability in the data for the main outcomes?	Yes	☐ 1
	No	☐ 0
In non-normally distributed data the inter-quartile range of results should be reported. In normally distributed data the standard error, standard deviation or confidence intervals should be reported. If the distribution of data is not described, it must be assumed that the estimates used were appropriate and the question should be answered 'yes'.		
8A Have all important adverse events that may be a consequence of the intervention been reported?	Yes	☐ 1
	No	☐ 0
This should be answered 'yes' if the study demonstrates that there was a comprehensive attempt to measure adverse events.		
9A Have the characteristics of subjects lost to follow-up been described?	Yes	☐ 1
	No	☐ 0
This should be answered 'yes' where there were no losses to follow-up or where losses to follow-up were so small that findings would be unaffected by their inclusion. This should be answered 'no' where a study does not report the number of subjects lost to the follow-up.		
10A Have the actual probability values been reported (e.g. 0.035 rather than <0.05) for the main outcomes except where the probability value is less than 0.001?	Yes	☐ 1
	No	☐ 0

External validity

The following criteria attempt to address the representativeness of the findings of the study and whether they may be generalised to the population (e.g. all nurses) from which the study subjects were derived.

11A Were the subjects asked to participate in the study representative of the entire population from which they were recruited? The study must identify the source population and describe how subjects were selected. Subjects would be representative if they comprised the entire source population, or a random sample. Where a study does not report the proportion of the source population from which the subjects are derived the question should be answered as 'unable to determine'.	Yes ☐ 1 No ☐ 0 Unable ☐ 0 to determine
12A Were those subjects who were prepared to participate representative of the entire population from which they were recruited? The proportion of those asked that agreed should be stated. Validation that the sample was representative would include demonstrating that the distribution of the main confounding factors was the same in the study sample and the source population.	Yes ☐ 1 No ☐ 0 Unable ☐ 0 to determine
13A Were the subjects, place and facilities where the study was set representative of the working environment? For the question to be answered 'yes' the study should demonstrate that the intervention was representative of that in use for the source population. The question should be answered 'no' if, for example, the intervention was done in a specialist centre unrepresentative of the hospitals where subjects would work. This means we cannot combine from different working environments – acute v. community.	Yes ☐ 1 No ☐ 0 Unable ☐ 0 to determine

Internal validity – bias

14A Was an attempt made to blind study subjects to the intervention they have received? For studies where the subjects would have no way of knowing which intervention they received, this should be answered 'yes'.	Yes ☐ 1 No ☐ 0 Unable ☐ 0 to determine
15A Was an attempt made to blind those measuring the main outcomes of the intervention?	Yes ☐ 1 No ☐ 0 Unable ☐ 0 to determine
16A If any of the results of the study were based on 'data dredging', was this made clear? Any analyses that had not been planned at the outset of the study should be clearly indicated. If no retrospective unplanned subgroup analyses were reported, then answer 'yes'.	Yes ☐ 1 No ☐ 0 Unable ☐ 0 to determine

17A In trials and cohort studies, do the analyses adjust for different lengths of follow-up of subjects; or in case–control studies, is the time period between the intervention and the outcome the same for cases and controls? Where follow-up was the same for all subjects the answer should be 'yes'. If different lengths of follow-up were adjusted the answer should be 'yes'. Studies where differences in follow-up are ignored should be answered 'no'.	Yes ☐ 1 No ☐ 0 Unable ☐ 0 to determine
18A Were the statistical tests used to assess the main outcomes appropriate? The statistical tests must be appropriate to the data. For example non-parametric methods should be used for small sample sizes. Where little statistical analysis has been undertaken but where there is no evidence of bias, the question should be answered 'yes'. If the distribution of the data (normal or not) is not described it must be assumed that the estimates used were appropriate and the question answered 'yes'.	Yes ☐ 1 No ☐ 0 Unable ☐ 0 to determine
19A Was compliance with the interventions(s) reliable? Where there was non-compliance (e.g. didn't use the equipment) or where there was contamination of one group, the question should be answered 'no'. For studies where the effect of any misclassification was likely to bias any association to the null, the question should be answered 'yes'.	Yes ☐ 1 No ☐ 0 Unable ☐ 0 to determine
20A Were the main outcome measures used accurate (valid and reliable)? For studies where the outcome measures are clearly described, the question should be answered 'yes'. For studies which refer to other work or that demonstrate the outcome measures are accurate, the question should be answered 'yes'.	Yes ☐ 1 No ☐ 0 Unable ☐ 0 to determine

Internal validity – confounding (selection bias)

21A Were the subjects in different groups (trial and cohort studies), or were the cases and controls (case–control studies) recruited from the same population? For example nurses for all comparison groups should be selected from the same hospital. The question should be answered 'unable to determine' for cohort groups and case–control studies where there is no information concerning the source of the workers included in the study.	Yes ☐ 1 No ☐ 0 Unable ☐ 0 to determine
22A Were study subjects in different intervention groups (trials and cohort studies) or were cases and controls (case–control studies) recruited over the same period of time? For a study that does not specify the time period over which subjects were recruited, the question should be answered as 'unable to determine'.	Yes ☐ 1 No ☐ 0 Unable ☐ 0 to determine

23A Were study subjects randomised to intervention groups?	Yes	☐ 1
Studies that state that subjects were randomised should be answered 'yes' except where method of randomisation would not ensure random allocation. For example alternate allocation would score 'no' because it is predictable.	No Unable to determine	☐ 0 ☐ 0

24A Was the randomisation assignment concealed from subjects until recruitment was complete and irrevocable?	Yes	☐ 1
All non-randomised studies should be answered 'no'.	No Unable to determine	☐ 0 ☐ 0

25A Was there adequate adjustment for confounding in the analysis from which the main findings were drawn?	Yes	☐ 1
The question should be answered 'no' if: the main conclusions of the study were based on intervention (or equipment used) rather than intentions at the outset. In non-randomised studies if the effect of the main confounders was not investigated or confounding was demonstrated but no adjustment was made in the final analysis the question should be answered 'no'.	No Unable to determine	☐ 0 ☐ 0

26A Were losses of subject follow-up taken into account?	Yes	☐ 1
If the number of subjects lost to follow-up is not reported then the question should be answered as 'unable to determine'. If the proportion lost to follow-up was too small to affect the main findings, the question should be answered 'yes'.	No Unable to determine	☐ 0 ☐ 0

Section B
Cohort/case–control studies

1B Is the hypothesis/aim/objective of the study clearly described?	Yes No	☐ 1 ☐ 0

2B Are the main outcomes to be measured clearly described in the Introduction or Methods section?	Yes No	☐ 1 ☐ 0
If the main outcomes are first mentioned in the Results section, the question should be answered 'no'.		

3B Sampling: are the characteristics of the subjects included in the study clearly described?	Yes No	☐ 1 ☐ 0
In cohort studies and trials, inclusion and/or exclusion criteria should be given. In case–control studies, a case definition and source for controls should be given.		

4B Are the factors of interest clearly described?	Yes No	☐ 1 ☐ 0
Equipment or changes in technique that are to be explored should be clearly described.		

5B Are the distributions of the principal confounders in each group of subjects to be compared clearly described?	Yes	☐ 2
(Confounding variable = an unforeseen and unaccounted for variable that jeopardises reliability and validity of an experiment outcome.)	Partially No	☐ 1 ☐ 0

6B Are the main findings of the study clearly described? Simple outcome data should be reported for all major findings so that the reader can check the major analyses and conclusions (see Question 18 for statistical tests).	Yes No	☐ 1 ☐ 0
7B Does the study provide estimates of the random variability in the data for the main outcomes? In non-normally distributed data the inter-quartile range of results should be reported. In normally distributed data the standard error, standard deviation or confidence intervals should be reported. If the distribution of data is not described, it must be assumed that the estimates used were appropriate and the question should be answered 'yes'.	Yes No	☐ 1 ☐ 0
8B Have all important adverse events that may be a consequence of the study been reported? This should be answered 'yes' if the study demonstrates that there was a comprehensive attempt to measure adverse events.	Yes No	☐ 1 ☐ 0
9B Have the characteristics of subjects lost to follow-up been described? This should be answered 'yes' where there were no losses to follow-up or where losses to follow-up were so small that findings would be unaffected by their inclusion. This should be answered 'no' where a study does not report the number of subjects lost to the follow-up.	Yes No	☐ 1 ☐ 0
10B Have the actual probability values been reported (e.g. 0.035 rather than <0.05) for the main outcomes except where the probability value is less than 0.001?	Yes No	☐ 1 ☐ 0

External validity

The following criteria attempt to address the representativeness of the findings of the study and whether they may be generalised to the population (e.g. all nurses) from which the study subjects were derived.

11B Were the subjects asked to participate in the study representative of the entire population from which they were recruited? The study must identify the source population and describe how subjects were selected. Subjects would be representative if they comprised the entire source population, or a random sample. Where a study does not report the proportion of the source population from which the subjects are derived the question should be answered as 'unable to determine'.	Yes No Unable to determine	☐ 1 ☐ 0 ☐ 0
12B Were those subjects who were prepared to participate representative of the entire population from which they were recruited? The proportion of those asked that agreed should be stated. Validation that the sample was representative would include demonstrating that the distribution of the main confounding factors was the same in the study sample and the source population.	Yes No Unable to determine	☐ 1 ☐ 0 ☐ 0

13B Were the place and facilities where the study was set representative of the working environment? The question should be answered 'no' if, for example, the study was done in a specialist centre unrepresentative of the general hospitals to which the study was generalised. This means we cannot combine from different working environments – acute v. community.	Yes ☐ 1 No ☐ 0 Unable ☐ 0 to determine

Internal validity – bias

15B Was an attempt made to blind those measuring the main outcomes?	Yes ☐ 1 No ☐ 0 Unable ☐ 0 to determine
16B If any of the results of the study were based on 'data dredging', was this made clear? Any analyses that had not been planned at the outset of the study should be clearly indicated. If no retrospective unplanned subgroup analyses were reported, then answer 'yes'.	Yes ☐ 1 No ☐ 0 Unable ☐ 0 to determine
17B Do the analyses adjust for different lengths of follow-up of subjects, or in case–control studies, is the time period the same for cases and controls? Where follow-up was the same for all subjects the answer should be 'yes'. If different lengths of follow-up were adjusted the answer should be 'yes'. Studies where differences in follow-up are ignored should be answered 'no'.	Yes ☐ 1 No ☐ 0 Unable ☐ 0 to determine
18B Were the statistical tests used to assess the main outcomes appropriate? The statistical tests must be appropriate to the data. For example non-parametric methods should be used for small sample sizes. Where little statistical analysis has been undertaken but where there is no evidence of bias, the question should be answered 'yes'. If the distribution of the data (normal or not) is not described it must be assumed that the estimates used were appropriate and the question answered 'yes'.	Yes ☐ 1 No ☐ 0 Unable ☐ 0 to determine
19B Was compliance with the investigation reliable? Where there was non-compliance (e.g. didn't use the equipment) or where there was contamination of one group, the question should be answered 'no'. For studies where the effect of any misclassification was likely to bias any association to the null, the question should be answered 'yes'.	Yes ☐ 1 No ☐ 0 Unable ☐ 0 to determine
20B Were the main outcome measures used accurate (valid and reliable)? For studies where the outcome measures are clearly described, the question should be answered 'yes'. For studies which refer to other work or that demonstrate the outcome measures are accurate, the question should be answered 'yes'.	Yes ☐ 1 No ☐ 0 Unable ☐ 0 to determine

Internal validity – confounding (selection bias)

21B Were the subjects in different groups or were the cases and controls recruited from the same population? For example nurses for all comparison groups should be selected from the same hospital. The question should be answered 'unable to determine' for cohort groups and case–control studies where there is no information concerning the source of the workers included in the study.	Yes No Unable to determine	☐ 1 ☐ 0 ☐ 0
22B Were study subjects in different groups or were cases and controls recruited over the same period of time? For a study that does not specify the time period over which subjects were recruited, the question should be answered as 'unable to determine'.	Yes No Unable to determine	☐ 1 ☐ 0 ☐ 0
25B Was there adequate adjustment for confounding in the analysis from which the main findings were drawn? In studies where the effect of the main confounders was not investigated or confounding was demonstrated but no adjustment was made in the final analysis the question should be answered 'no'.	Yes No Unable to determine	☐ 1 ☐ 0 ☐ 0
26B Were losses of subject follow-up taken into account? If the number of subjects lost to follow-up is not reported then the question should be answered as 'unable to determine'. If the proportion lost to follow-up was too small to affect the main findings, the question should be answered 'yes'.	Yes No Unable to determine	☐ 1 ☐ 0 ☐ 0

Section C
Cross-sectional studies, inc. surveys

1C Is the hypothesis/aim/objective of the study clearly described?	Yes No	☐ 1 ☐ 0
2C Are the main outcomes to be measured clearly described in the Introduction or Methods section? If the main outcomes are first mentioned in the Results section, the question should be answered 'no'.	Yes No	☐ 1 ☐ 0
2Ci Was a standardised questionnaire used? If they included questionnaire piloting with a clear description of the testing procedures and a description of any changes and subsequent pilot: answer 'yes', otherwise answer 'no'.	Yes No	☐ 1 ☐ 0
3C Sampling: Are the characteristics of the subjects included in the study clearly described? In cohort studies and trials, inclusion and/or exclusion criteria should be given. In case–control studies, a case definition and source for controls should be given.	Yes No	☐ 1 ☐ 0

5C Are the distributions of the principal confounders in each group of subjects to be compared clearly described? (Confounding variable = an unforeseen and unaccounted for variable that jeopardises reliability and validity of an experiment outcome.)	Yes ☐ 2 Partially ☐ 1 No ☐ 0
6C Are the main findings of the study clearly described? Simple outcome data should be reported for all major findings so that the reader can check the major analyses and conclusions (see Question 18 for statistical tests).	Yes ☐ 1 No ☐ 0
7C Does the study provide estimates of the random variability in the data for the main outcomes? In non-normally distributed data the inter-quartile range of results should be reported. In normally distributed data the standard error, standard deviation or confidence intervals should be reported. If the distribution of data is not described, it must be assumed that the estimates used were appropriate and the question should be answered 'yes'.	Yes ☐ 1 No ☐ 0
8C Have all important adverse events that may be a consequence of the study been reported? This should be answered 'yes' if the study demonstrates that there was a comprehensive attempt to measure adverse events.	Yes ☐ 1 No ☐ 0
9C Have the characteristics of subjects lost to follow-up been described? This should be answered 'yes' where there were no losses to follow-up or where losses to follow-up were so small that findings would be unaffected by their inclusion. This should be answered 'no' where a study does not report the number of subjects lost to the follow-up.	Yes ☐ 1 No ☐ 0
10C Have the actual probability values been reported (e.g. 0.035 rather than <0.05) for the main outcomes except where the probability value is less than 0.001?	Yes ☐ 1 No ☐ 0

External validity

The following criteria attempt to address the representativeness of the findings of the study and whether they may be generalised to the population (e.g. all nurses) from which the study subjects were derived.

11C Were the subjects asked to participate in the study representative of the entire population from which they were recruited? The study must identify the source population and describe how subjects were selected. Subjects would be representative if they comprised the entire source population, or a random sample. Where a study does not report the proportion of the source population from which the subjects are derived the question should be answered as 'unable to determine'.	Yes ☐ 1 No ☐ 0 Unable ☐ 0 to determine

12C Were those subjects who were prepared to participate representative of the entire population from which they were recruited? The proportion of those asked that agreed should be stated. Validation that the sample was representative would include demonstrating that the distribution of the main confounding factors was the same in the study sample and the source population.	Yes ☐ 1 No ☐ 0 Unable ☐ 0 to determine
13C Were the subjects, place and facilities where the study was set representative of the working environment? The question should be answered 'no' if, for example, the study was done in a specialist centre unrepresentative of the general hospitals to which the study was generalised. This means we cannot combine from different working environments – acute v. community.	Yes ☐ 1 No ☐ 0 Unable ☐ 0 to determine

Internal validity – bias

15C Was an attempt made to blind those measuring the main outcomes?	Yes ☐ 1 No ☐ 0 Unable ☐ 0 to determine
16C If any of the results of the study were based on 'data dredging', was this made clear? Any analyses that had not been planned at the outset of the study should be clearly indicated. If no retrospective unplanned subgroup analyses were reported, then answer 'yes'.	Yes ☐ 1 No ☐ 0 Unable ☐ 0 to determine
18C Were the statistical tests used to assess the main outcomes appropriate? The statistical tests must be appropriate to the data. For example non-parametric methods should be used for small sample sizes. Where little statistical analysis has been undertaken but where there is no evidence of bias, the question should be answered 'yes'. If the distribution of the data (normal or not) is not described it must be assumed that the estimates used were appropriate and the question answered 'yes'.	Yes ☐ 1 No ☐ 0 Unable ☐ 0 to determine
20C Were the main outcome measures used accurate (valid and reliable)? For studies where the outcome measures are clearly described, the question should be answered 'yes'. For studies which refer to other work or that demonstrate the outcome measures are accurate, the question should be answered 'yes'.	Yes ☐ 1 No ☐ 0 Unable ☐ 0 to determine

Internal validity – confounding (selection bias)

21C Were the subjects recruited from the same population? For example all nurses in a study population should be selected from the same hospital. The question should be answered 'unable to determine' where there is no information concerning the source of the study population.	Yes ☐ 1 No ☐ 0 Unable ☐ 0 to determine
22C Were study subjects recruited over a defined period of time? For a study that does not specify the time period over which subjects were recruited, the question should be answered as 'unable to determine'.	Yes ☐ 1 No ☐ 0 Unable ☐ 0 to determine
25C Was there adequate adjustment for confounding in the analysis from which the main findings were drawn? In studies where the effect of the main confounders was not investigated or confounding was demonstrated but no adjustment was made in the final analysis the question should be answered 'no'.	Yes ☐ 1 No ☐ 0 Unable ☐ 0 to determine
26C Were losses of subject follow-up taken into account? If the number of subjects lost to follow-up is not reported then the question should be answered as 'unable to determine'. If the proportion lost to follow-up was too small to affect the main findings, the question should be answered 'yes'. In a survey there should be reference to questionnaire reminders.	Yes ☐ 1 No ☐ 0 Unable ☐ 0 to determine

Section D
Case series

1D Is the hypothesis/aim/objective of the study clearly described?	Yes ☐ 1 No ☐ 0
3D Sampling: are the characteristics of the subjects included in the study clearly described? In cohort studies and trials, inclusion and/or exclusion criteria should be given. In case–control studies, a case definition and source for controls should be given.	Yes ☐ 1 No ☐ 0
6D Are the main findings of the study clearly described? Simple outcome data should be reported for all major findings so that the reader can check the major analyses and conclusions (see Question 18 for statistical tests).	Yes ☐ 1 No ☐ 0
9D Have the characteristics of subjects lost to the series been described? This should be answered 'yes' where there were no losses or where losses were so small that findings would be unaffected by their inclusion. This should be answered 'no' where a study does not report the number of subjects.	Yes ☐ 1 No ☐ 0
10D Have the actual probability values been reported (e.g. 0.035 rather than <0.05) for the main outcomes except where the probability value is less than 0.001?	Yes ☐ 1 No ☐ 0

External validity

The following criteria attempt to address the representativeness of the findings of the study and whether they may be generalised to the population (e.g. all nurses) from which the study subjects were derived.

11D Were the subjects asked to participate in the study representative of the entire population from which they were recruited? The study must identify the source population and describe how subjects were selected. Subjects would be representative if they comprised the entire source population, or a random sample. Where a study does not report the proportion of the source population from which the subjects are derived the question should be answered as 'unable to determine'.	Yes ☐ 1 No ☐ 0 Unable ☐ 0 to determine
12D Were those subjects who were prepared to participate representative of the entire population from which they were recruited? The proportion of those asked that agreed should be stated. Validation that the sample was representative would include demonstrating that the distribution of the main confounding factors was the same in the study sample and the source population.	Yes ☑ 1 No ☐ 0 Unable ☐ 0 to determine
13D Were the place and facilities where the study was set representative of the working environment? The question should be answered 'no' if, for example, the study was done in a specialist centre unrepresentative of the general hospitals to which the study was generalised. This means we cannot combine from different working environments – acute v. community.	Yes ☐ 1 No ☐ 0 Unable ☐ 0 to determine

Internal validity – bias

18D Were the statistical tests used to assess the main outcomes appropriate? The statistical tests must be appropriate to the data. For example non-parametric methods should be used for small sample sizes. Where little statistical analysis has been undertaken but where there is no evidence of bias, the question should be answered 'yes'. If the distribution of the data (normal or not) is not described it must be assumed that the estimates used were appropriate and the question answered 'yes'.	Yes ☐ 1 No ☐ 0 Unable ☐ 0 to determine
20D Were the main outcome measures used accurate (valid and reliable)? For studies where the outcome measures are clearly described, the question should be answered 'yes'. For studies which refer to other work or that demonstrate the outcome measures are accurate, the question should be answered 'yes'.	Yes ☐ 1 No ☑ 0 Unable ☐ 0 to determine

Internal validity – confounding (selection bias)

21D Were the subjects described recruited from the same population? For example nurses for all comparison groups should be selected from the same hospital. The question should be answered 'unable to determine' where there is no information concerning the source of the subjects included in the study.	Yes ☐ 1 No ☐ 0 Unable ☐ 0 to determine
22D Were study subjects recruited over a defined period of time? For a study that does not specify the time period over which subjects were recruited, the question should be answered as 'unable to determine'.	Yes ☐ 1 No ☐ 0 Unable ☐ 0 to determine
26D Were losses of subject follow-up taken into account? If the number of subjects lost is not reported then the question should be answered as 'unable to determine'. If the proportion lost was too small to affect the main findings, the question should be answered 'yes'.	Yes ☐ 1 No ☐ 0 Unable ☐ 0 to determine

Section E
Questions about qualitative studies

27 Is the hypothesis/aim/objective of the study clearly described?	Yes ☐ 1 No ☐ 0
28 Are the research methods appropriate to the question being asked?	Yes ☐ 1 No ☐ 0
29 Was the qualitative method that was used made clear in the aims of the study?	Yes ☐ 1 No ☐ 0
30 Is there a clear connection to an existing body of knowledge/ wider theoretical framework?	Yes ☐ 1 No ☐ 0
31 Is the context for the research adequately described and accounted for?	Yes ☐ 1 No ☐ 0
32 Are the criteria for, and approach to, sample selection, data collection and analysis described clearly and systematically applied?	Yes ☐ 1 No ☐ 0
33 Does the paper describe the sample in terms of gender, ethnicity, social class, etc. (if appropriate)?	Yes ☐ 1 No ☐ 0
34 Was the sample appropriate?	Yes ☐ 1 No ☐ 0
35 Were the processes of fieldwork and the means of data collection described adequately?	Yes ☐ 1 No ☐ 0

36 Is the relationship between the researcher and the researched considered and have the latter been fully informed?	Yes	☐ 1
	No	☐ 0
37 Is sufficient consideration given to how findings are derived from the data and how the validity of the findings were tested (negative examples, member checking)?	Yes	☐ 1
	No	☐ 0
38 Has evidence for and against the researcher's interpretation been considered?	Yes	☐ 1
	No	☐ 0
39 Are the findings systematically reported and is sufficient original evidence reported to justify relationships between evidence and conclusions?	Yes	☐ 1
	No	☐ 0

EXCLUDED STUDIES

NO TASK, EQUIPMENT OR INTERVENTION

Abidi, D. and Gilbert, R. (1995) 'L'ergonomie dans le processus de reconception d'un lève-personne protatif sur rail au plafond', *Proceedings of the 27th Annual Congress of the Human Factors Association of Canada,* Canada: Human Factors Association, 205–8.

Aickin, C. (1991) 'Forward trunk inclination in physiotherapy work', in Queinnec, Y. and Daniellou, F. (eds) *Designing for Everyone, Proceedings of the 11th congress of the IEA, Paris,* Taylor & Francis, 3: 13–14.

Alavosius, M., Sulzer-Azaroff, B. (1985) 'An on-the-job method to evaluate patient lifting technique', *Applied Ergonomics* 16 (4): 307–11.

Alexandre, N.M. and Benatti, M.C. (1998) 'Occupational accidents involving the spine: study on nurses at a university hospital', *Revista Latino-Americana de Enfermagem* 6: 65–72.

Ando, S., Ono, Y., Shimaoka, M., Hiruta, S., Hattori, Y., Hori, F. and Takeuchi, Y. (2000) 'Associations of self estimated workloads with musculoskeletal symptoms amount hospital nurses', *Occupational & Environmental Medicine* 57: 211–16.

Atkinson, F.I. (1992) 'Experiences of informal carers providing nursing support for disabled dependants', *Journal of Advanced Nursing* 17: 835–40.

Baldasseroni, A., Tartaglia, R., Sgarrella, C. and Carnevale, F. (1998) 'Frequency of lumbago in a cohort of nursing students', *Giornale Italiano di Medicina del Lavoro* 89: 245–53.

Baty, D. and Stubbs, D.A. (1987) 'Postural stress in geriatric nursing', *International Journal of Nursing Studies* 24 (4): 339–44.

Benyon, C., Burke, J., Doran, D. and Nevill, A. (2000) 'Effects of activity-rest schedules on physiological strain and spinal load in hospital-based porters', *Ergonomics* 43(10): 1763–70.

Best, M. and Lyons, S. (1991) 'Manutention – a new handle on backs in Australia', in Queinnec, Y. and Daniellou, F. (eds) *Designing for Everyone, Proceedings of the 11th congress of the IEA, Paris,* Taylor & Francis, 200–3.

Biering-Sorensen, F., Vejerslev, L.O. and Gyntelberg, F. (1981) 'Reported back injuries caused by manual transport and lifting among a hospital staff', *Ugeskrift for Laeger* 143: 947–51.

Bobick, T.G., Pizatella, T.J., Hsiao, H. and Amendola, A.A. (1995) 'Job-design characteristics that contribute to workplace-related musculoskeletal injuries: considerations for health care professionals', *Orthopaedic Physical Therapy Clinics of North America* 4: 385.

Boden, M. (1999) 'Infection control in moving and handling', *Professional Nurse* 14 (16): 387–9.

Bonatti, D., Merseburger, A., Bombana, S., Gisser, G. and Paternoster, D. (1999) 'Assessment of exposure to risk due to manual lifting of patients and results of clinical studies in geriatric residences in the Mantua area', *Giornale Italiano di Medicina del Lavoro* 90: 276–90.

Bordini, L., De Vito, G., Molteni, G. and Boccardi, S. (1999) 'Epidemiology of musculoskeletal alterations due to biochemical overload of the spine in manual lifting of patients', *Giornale Italiano di Medicina del Lavoro* 90: 103–16.

Bork, B.E., Cook, T.M., Rosecrance, J.C., Engelhardt, K.A., Thomason, M.J., Wauford, I.J. and Worley, R.K. (1996) 'Work-related musculoskeletal disorders among physical therapists', *Physical Therapy* 76 (8): 827–35.

Brown, L. (1988) 'They don't look like weight lifters ... nurses and back injury', *New Zealand Hospital*, 22–4.

Bru, E., Mykletun, R.J. and Svebak, S. (1994) 'Assessment of musculoskeletal and other health complaints in female hospital staff', *Applied Ergonomics* 25 (2): 101–5.

Brulin, C., Gerdle, B., Granlund, B., Hoog, J., Knutson, A. and Sundelin, G. (1988) 'Physical and psychosocial work-related risk factors associated with musculoskeletal symptoms among home care personnel', *Scandinavian Journal of Caring Sciences* 12: 104–10.

Buckle, P. (1987) 'Epidemiological aspects of back pain within the nursing profession', *International Journal of Nursing Studies* 24 (4): 310–24.

Burton, A.K., Symonds, T.L., Zinzen, E., Tillotson, K.M., Caboor, D., Van Roy, P. and Clarys, J.P. (1997) 'Is ergonomic intervention alone sufficient to limit musculoskeletal problems in nurses?' *Occupational Medicine* 47 (1): 25–32.

Busse, M. and Bridger, R.S. (1997) 'Cost benefits of ergonomic intervention in a hospital. A preliminary study using Oxenburg's productivity model', *Curationis* 20 (3): 54–8.

Busse, M. and Geal, L. (1999) 'The pitfalls of stroke rehabilitation: access to care', *Nursing & Residential Care* 1 (6): 324–8.

Camerino, D., Molteni, G., Capietti, M., Molinari, M., Cotroneo, L. *et al.* (1999) 'The prevention of risk due to the manual lifting of patients: the psychosocial component', *Giornale Italiano di Medicina del Lavoro* 90 (2): 412–27.

Capodaglio, E.M., Capodaglio, P. and Bazzini, G. (1999) 'Multifactorial ergonomic evaluation of the hospital nursing activity in assisting not self-sufficient patients', *Giornale Italiano di Medicina del Lavoro* 21 (2): 134–9.

Cedercreutz, G., Videman, T., Tola, S. and Asp, S. (1987) 'Individual risk factors of the back among applicants to a nursing school', *Ergonomics* 30 (2): 269–72.

Coggan, C. and Roberts, I. (1994) 'Prevalence of back injuries among nurses', *New Zealand Medical Journal*, 306–9.

Cooper, J.E., Tate, R.B. and Yassi, A. (1998) 'Components of initial and residual disability after back injury in nurses', *Spine* 23: 2118–22.

Counsell, A. (1994) 'Mind your back', *Journal of Community Nursing* (December), 8–9.

Cowell, R. and Shuttleworth, A. (1988) 'Equipment for moving and handling patients', *Professional Nurse* 14: 123–30.

Cox, T.R. (1993) 'Nursing personnel accidents and their causes in a veterans affairs hospital', *Applied Occupational & Environmental Hygiene* 8 (8): 703–7.

Cromie, J.E., Robertson, V.J. and Best, M.O. (2000) 'Work-related musculoskeletal disorders in physical therapists: prevalence, security, risks, and responses', *Physical Therapy* 80: 336–51.

Cromie, J.E., Robertson, V.J. and Best, M.O. (2001) 'Occupational health and safety in physiotherapy: guidelines for practice', *Australian Journal of Physiotherapy* 47: 43–51.

Dehlin, O. and Berg, S. (1977) 'Back symptoms and psychological perception of work', *Scandinavian Journal of Rehabilitation Medicine* 9: 61–5.

Dehlin, O. and Jäderberg, E. (1982) 'Perceived exertion during patient lifts', *Scandinavian Journal of Rehabilitation Medicine* 14: 11–20.

Donnelly, C. (2000) 'Teaching the neuromuscular approach to efficient handling and moving', in McCabe, P., Hanson, M. and Robertson, S. (eds) *Contemporary Ergonomics,* London: Taylor & Francis, 255–9.

Eckles, K. (1993) 'Back problems among diagnostic radiographers', *Radiography Today* 59 (673): 17–20.

Elert, J., Brulin, C., Gerdle, B. and Johansson, H. (1992) 'Mechanical performance level of continuous contraction and muscle pain symptoms in home care personnel', *Scandinavian Journal of Rehabilitation Medicine* 24 (3): 141–50.

Ellis, B.E. (1993) 'Moving and handling patients: an evaluation of current training for physiotherapy students', *Physiotherapy* 79 (5): 323–6.

Engels, J.A., Landeweerd, J. and Kant, Y. (1994) 'An OWAS-based analysis of nurses' working postures', *Ergonomics* 37 (5): 909–19.

Engels, J.A., Van der Gulden, J.W.J. and Senden, T.F. (1997) 'Prevention of musculo-skeletal complaints in nursing: aims, approach and content of an ergonomic-educational programme', *Safety Science* 27 (2/3): 141–8.

Engels, J.A., Van der Gulden, J.W.J., Senden T.F., Hertog, C.A.W.M., Kolk, J.J. and Binkhorst. R.A. (1994) 'Physical work load and its assessment among the nursing staff in nursing homes', *Journal of Occupational Medicine* 36 (3): 338–45.

Engels, J.A., Van der Gulden, J.W.J., Senden, T.F. and van't Hof B. (1996) 'Work related risk factors for musculoskeletal complaints in the nursing profession: results of a questionnaire survey', *Occupational & Environmental Medicine* 53: 636–41.

Engkvist, I.L., Hagberg, M., Hjelm, E.W., Menckel, E. and Ekenvall, L. (1998) 'The accident process preceding over-exertion back injuries in nursing personnel: PROSA study group', *Scandinavian Journal of Work, Environment & Health* 24: 467–75.

Engkvist, I.L., Hagberg, M., Wigaeus-Hjelm, E., Menckel, E. and Ekenvall, L. (1995) 'Interview protocols and ergonomics checklist for analysing overexertion back accidents among nursing personnel', *Applied Ergonomics* 26 (3): 213–20.

Engkvist, I.L., Hjelm, E.W., Hagberg, M., Menckel, E. and Ekenvall, L. (2000) 'Risk indicators for reported over-exertion back injuries among female nursing personnel', *Epidemiology* 11 (5): 519–22.

Engkvist, I.L., Hagberg, A., Lindén, A. and Malker, B. (1992) 'Over-exertion back accidents among nurses' aides in Sweden', *Safety Science* 15: 97–108.

Ersson, A., Lundberg, M., Wramby, C.O. and Svensson, H. (1999) 'Extrication of entrapped victims from motor vehicle accidents: the crew concept', *European Journal of Emergency Medicine* 6: 341–7.

Estryn-Behar, M., Kaminski, M., Peigne, E., Maillard, M.F., Pelletier, A., Berthier, C., Delaporte, M.F., Paoli, M.C. and Leroux, J.M. (1990) 'Strenuous working conditions and musculo-skeletal disorders among female hospital workers', *International Archives of Occupational and Environmental Health*. 62: 47–57.

Ferguson, D. (1970) 'Strain injuries in hospital employees', *The Medical Journal of Australia,* 376–9.

Fieret, G. (1983) 'Ergonomics and nursing', *Tijdschrift voor Ziekenverpleging* 36: 661–5.

Fjordbo, M. (1994) 'Work environment – there will be two with a lifting injury', *Sygeplejersken* 94: 40–1.

Fortuna, R. and Ricci, M.G. (1999) 'Manual lifting of patients: results of assessment of exposure to specific risk and of clinical studies in a rehabilitation centre', *Giornale Italiano di Medicina del Lavoro* 90 (2): 317–29.

French, P., Flora, L.F.W., Ping, L.S., Bo, L.K. and Rita, W.H.Y. (1997) 'The prevalence and cause of occupational back pain in Hong Kong registered nurses', *Journal of Advanced Nursing* 26: 380–8.

Frigo, C. (1999) 'Instrumental investigations in laboratories specialized in assessing disk overload in hospital workers', *Giornale Italiano di Medicina del Lavoro* 90 (2): 117–30.

Fuortes, L.J., Shi, Y., Zhang, M., Zwerling, C. and Schootman, M. (1994) 'Epidemiology of back injury in university hospital nurses from review of workers' compensation records and a case–control survey', *Journal of Occupational Medicine* 36 (9): 1022–6.

Garg, A. (1993) 'What basis exists for training workers in "correct" lifting techniques', in Marras, W.S., Karwowski, W., Smith, J.L. and Pacholski, L. (eds) *The Ergonomics of Manual Work: Proceedings of the IEA world conference, Poland 14–17 June*, London: Taylor & Francis, 89–91.

Garrett, B., Singiser, D. and Banks, S.M. (1992) 'Back injuries among nursing personnel: the relationship of personal characteristics, risk factors, and nursing practices', *AAOHN Journal* 40 (11): 510–16.

Gerdle, B., Brulin, C., Elert, J. and Granlund, B. (1994) 'Factors interacting with perceived work-related complaints in the musculoskeletal system among home care service personnel', *Scandinavian Journal of Rehabilitation Medicine* 26: 51–8.

Gladman, G. (1993) 'Back pain in student nurses – the mature factor', *Occupational Health*, 47–51.

Goldman, R.H., Jarrard, M.R., Kim, R., Loomis, S. and Atkins, E.H. (2000) 'Prioritizing back injury risk in hospital employees: application and comparison of different injury rates', *Journal of Occupational & Environmental Medicine* 42 (6): 645–52.

Gordon, K. (1991) 'Devising a back pain prevention package', *Nursing Standard* 6 (4): 25–8.

Graves, R.J., Morales, A. and Seaton, A. (1995) 'Assessing risk in nursing activities – can patient handling assessments be improved?' in Robertson, S. (ed.) *Contemporary Ergonomics: Proceedings of the Ergonomics Society 1995 Annual Conference*, London: Taylor & Francis, 385–91.

Green, S. and Gillett, A. (1998) 'Caring for patients with morbid obesity in hospital', *British Journal of Nursing* 7 (13): 785–92.

Greenwood, J.G. (1986) 'Back injuries can be reduced with worker training, reinforcement', *Occupational Health & Safety*, May: 26–9.

Grisbrooke, J. and Pearce, J. (1999) 'Moving and handing education for student OTs and physiotherapists', *British Journal of Therapy and Rehabilitation* 6 (5): 233–8.

Gundewall, B., Lijequist, M. and Hansson, T. (1993) 'Primary prevention of back symptoms and absence from work. A prospective randomised study among hospital employees', *Spine* 18 (5): 587–94.

Harber, P., Billet, E., Lew, M. and Horan, M. (1987) 'Importance of non-patient transfer activities in nursing-related back pain', *Journal of Occupational Medicine* 29 (12): 967–74.

Harber, P., Billet, E., Shimozaki, S. and Vojtecky, M. (1988) 'Occupational back pain of nurses: special problems and prevention', *Applied Ergonomics* 19 (3): 219–24.

Harber, P., Billet, E., Vojtecky, M., Rosenthal, E., Shimozaki, S. and Horan, M. (1988) 'Nurses' beliefs about cause and prevention of occupational back pain', *Journal of Occupational Medicine* 30 (10): 797–800.

Harvey, J. (1985) 'A survey of staff attitudes towards lifting patients and objects and the causes of back pain at Witney Community Hospital', Oxfordshire Health Unit: Centre for Health Promotion and Education.

Harvey, J. (1987) 'Back to the drawing board', *Nursing Times* 88: 47–8.

Heap, D.C. (1987) 'Low back injuries in nursing staff', *Journal of the Society of Occupational Medicine* 37: 66–9.

Hefferin, E.A. and Hill, B.J. (1976) 'Analysing nursing's work-related injuries', *American Journal of Nursing* 76 (6): 924–7.

Hignett, S. (1994) 'Physiotherapists and the manual handling operations regulations', *Physiotherapy* 80 (7): 446–7.

Hignett, S. (1994) 'Shifting the emphasis in patient handling', *Occupational Health* 130 (46): 127–8.

Hignett, S. (1994) 'Using computerised OWAS for postural analysis of nursing work', in Robertson, S. (ed.) *Contemporary Ergonomics. Proceedings of the Ergonomics Society Annual Conference,* London: Taylor & Francis, 253–8.

Hignett, S. (1995) 'Fitting the work to the physiotherapist', *Physiotherapy* 81 (9): 549–52.

Hignett, S. (1996) 'Postural analysis of nursing work', *Applied Ergonomics* 27 (3): 171–6.

Ho, S-T., Au Yeung, B., Au, G., Huang, H. and Ko, F. (1997) 'Study of back pain amongst nurses', *The Hong Kong Nursing Journal* 33 (2): 5–11.

Hogya, P.T. and Ellis, L. (1990) 'Evaluation of the injury profile of personnel in a busy urban system', *American Journal of Emergency Medicine* 8 (4): 308–9.

Hollingdale, R. (1997) 'Back pain in nursing and associated factors: a study', *Nursing Standard* 11 (39): 35–8.

Hoover, S.A. (1973) 'Job-related back injuries in a hospital', *American Journal of Nursing* 73 (12): 2078–9.

Jansen, J.P., Burdorf, A. and van der Beek, A.J. (2000) 'Lumbar posture during work among nurses and office workers and the relation to back problems: statistical analysis of angle-vs-time data', *Proceedings of the IEA2000/HFES 2000 Congress,* The Human Factors and Ergonomics Society, California: Santa Monica, 5: 465–568.

Jensen, R.C. (1985) 'Events that trigger disabling back pain among nurses', in *Proceedings of Human Factors Society 29th Annual meeting,* The Human Factors Society, California: Santa Monica, 799–801.

Jensen, R.C. (1987) 'Disabling back injuries among nursing personnel: research needs and justification', *Research in Nursing & Health* 10: 29–38.

Jensen, R.C. (1987) 'Low back pain and back injury among health care workers', *Occupational Hazards to Health Care Workers, American Conference of Governmental Industrial Hygienists,* 41–50.

Jensen, R.C. (1987) 'Epidemiologic studies of the back pain problems of nursing personnel – the need for consistency in future studies', *Trends in Ergonomics/Human Factors* IV, Holland: Elsevier Science Publishers B.V., 803–9.

Jensen, R.C. (1990) 'Back injuries among nursing personnel related to exposure', *Applied Occupational and Environmental Hygiene* 5: 38–45.

Jones, C. (1992) 'A systems approach to the prevention of back injuries among nursing personnel in critical care units', *Kentucky Nurse* 40 (3): 18.

Jones, J A.R., Cockcroft, A. and Richardson, B. (1999) 'The ability of non-ergonomists in the health care setting to make manual handling risk assessments and implement changes', *Applied Ergonomics* 30: 159–66.

Jorgensen, S., Hein, H.O. and Gyntelberg, G. (1994) 'Heavy lifting at work and risk of genital prolapse and herniated lumbar disc in assistant nurses', *Occupational Medicine* 44: 47–9.

Josephson, M. and Vingard, E. (1998) 'Workplace factors and care seeking for low-back pain among female nursing personnel', *Scandinavian Journal of Work, Environment & Health* 24: 465–72.

Josephson, M., Lagerström, M., Hagberg, M. and Hjelm, E.W. (1997) 'Musculoskeletal symptoms and job strain among nursing personnel: a study over a three year period', *Occupational and Environmental Medicine* 54: 681–5.

Jozwiak, Z.W. and Gadzicka, E. (1993) 'Biomechanical analysis of work postures of operating room staff', in Marras, W.S., Karwowski, W., Smith, J.L. and Pacholski, L. (eds)

'The Ergonomics of Manual Work', *Proceedings of the IEA world conference*, London: Taylor & Francis, 241–4.

Kilgariff, C. and Best, M. (1999) 'An investigation of manual handling training in Victorian health education programs', *Journal of Occupational Health & Safety – Australia & New Zealand* 15 (5): 475–81.

Kjellberg, K., Johnsson, C., Proper, K., Olsson, E. and Hagberg, M. (2000) 'An observation instrument for assessment of work technique in patient transfer tasks', *Applied Ergonomics* 31: 139–50.

Klaber Moffett, J.A., Hughes, G.I. and Griffiths, P. (1993) 'A longitudinal study of low back pain in student nurses', *International Journal of Nursing Studies* 30: 197–212.

Kneafsey, R. (2000) 'The effect of occupational socialization on nurses' patient handling practices', *Journal of Clinical Nursing* 9: 585–93.

Laflamme, L. (1998) 'Falls among Swedish nurses and nursing auxiliaries: types of injuries and their relation to age over time', *Work* 10: 147–55.

Lagerström, M., Wenemark, M., Hagberg, M. and Hjelm, E.W. (1995) 'Occupational and individual factors related to musculoskeletal symptoms in five body regions among Swedish nursing personnel', *International Archives of Occupational and Environmental Health* 68: 27–35.

Lagerström, M., Hansson, T. and Hagberg, M. (1998) 'Work-related low-back problems in nursing', *Scandinavian Journal of Work, Environment & Health* 24 (6): 449–64.

Landeweerd, J.A. and Kant, I. (1996) 'Working postures and physical load of ambulance nurses', *Advances in Applied Ergonomics*, 941–4.

Larese, F. and Fiorito, A. (1994) 'Musculoskeletal disorders in hospital nurses: a comparison between two hospitals', *Ergonomics* 37 (7): 1205–11.

Lee, Y.H. and Chiou, W.K. (1995) 'Ergonomic analysis of working posture in nursing personnel: example of modified Ovako working analysis system application', *Research in Nursing & Health* 18: 67–75.

Leyshon, G.E. and Francis, H.W.S. (1975) 'Lifting injuries in ambulance crews', *Public Health* 89: 71–5.

Lortie, M. (1987) 'Structural analysis of occupational accidents affecting orderlies in a geriatric hospital', *Journal of Occupational Medicine* 29 (5): 437–44.

Love, C. (1995) 'Managing manual handling in clinical situations', *Nursing Times* 95: 38–9.

Love, C. (1997) 'Lifting injury: a study of the occupational health perspective', *Nursing Standard* 11 (26): 33–8.

Love, C. (1997) 'A Delphi study examining standards for patient handling', *Nursing Standard* 11 (45): 34–8.

MacDonald, H., Vander Doelen, J.A. and Frauts, J. (1989) 'Ergonomic issues related to patient lifting', *Occupational Health in Ontario* 10 (1): 10–22.

Mandel, J.H. and Lohman, W. (1987) 'Low back pain in nurses: the relative importance of medical history, work factors, exercise and demographics', *Research in Nursing & Health* 10: 165–70.

Mandelstam, M. (2001) 'Safe use of disability equipment and manual handling: legal aspects – part 2, manual handling', *British Journal of Occupational Therapy* 64 (2): 73–80.

Marchi, T., Lorusso, A., Boetner, E. and Magarotto, G. (1993) 'Frequency of spinal disorders in operating theatre staff', *Giornale Italiano di Medicina del Lavoro* 84: 108–14.

Massironi, F., Mian, P., Olivato, D. and Bacis, M. (1999) 'Exposure to risk due to manual lifting of patients and results of clinical studies in four hospitals in northern Italy', *Giornale Italiano di Medicina del Lavoro* 90: 341.

Meittunen, E.J., Matzke, K. and Sobczak, S.C. (1999) 'Identification of risk factors for a challenging ergonomic issue: the patient transfer', *Journal of Healthcare Safety Compliance and Infection Control*, 9–19.

Menoni, O., Battevi, N., Ricci, M.G. and Occhipinti, E. (2000) 'Methods of exposure assessment of patient handling tasks: a new risk index (MAPO)', *Proceedings of the IEA2000/HFES 2000 Congress*, The Human Factors and Ergonomics Society, California: Santa Monica, 5: 789–92.

Meyer, J.D. and Muntaner, C. (1999) 'Injuries in home healthcare workers: an analysis of occupational morbidity from a state compensation database', *American Journal of Industrial Medicine* 35: 295–301.

Miller, S.D. and O'Brien, J.E. (1991) 'Prevalence of back pain among radiation therapists', *Radiologic Technology* 62 (6): 461–7.

Moens, G.F., Dohogne, T., Jacques, P. and van Helshoecht, P. (1993) 'Back pain and its correlates among workers in family care', *Occupational Medicine* 43: 78–84.

Morlock, M.M., Bonin, V., Deuretzbacher, G., Muller, G., Honl, M. and Schneider, E. (2000) 'Determination of the in vivo loading of the lumbar spine with a new approach directly at the workplace – first results for nurses', *Clinical Biomechanics* 15: 549–58.

Mucha, C. and Winkler, J. (1995) 'Back-school for nursing staff', *Rehabilitacia* 28: 29.

Myers, A., Jensen, R.C., Nestor, D. and Rattiner, J. (1993) Low back injuries among home health aides compared with hospital nursing aides', *Home Health Care Services Quarterly* 14 (2): 149–55.

Newsom, J.A. (1997) 'Working towards a lift-free hospital injury prevention in a long-stay care – the physiotherapist's special role', *NZ Journal of Physiotherapy*: 29–31.

Nicholls, J.A. (1997) 'Patient handling training and work-related back pain', *British Journal of Therapy & Rehabilitation* 4 (8): 429–34.

Ono, Y., Lagerström, M., Hagberg, M., Linden, A. and Malker, B. (1995) 'Reports of work related musculoskeletal injury among home care service workers compared with nursery school workers and the general population of employed women in Sweden', *Occupational and Environmental Medicine* 5: 686–93.

Owen, B.D. (1985) 'The lifting process and back injury in hospital nursing personnel', *Western Journal of Nursing Research* 7: 445–59.

Owen, B.D. (1986) 'Personal characteristics important to back injury', *Rehabilitation Nursing* 11 (4): 12–16.

Owen, B.D. and Damron, C.F. (1984) 'Personal characteristics and back injury among hospital nursing personnel', *Research in Nursing & Health* 7: 305–13.

Owen, B.D. (1989) 'The magnitude of low-back problems in nursing', *Western Journal of Nursing Research* 11 (2): 234–42.

Panciera, D., Menoni, O., Ricci, M.G. and Occhipinti, E. (1999) 'Criteria for choice of aids for patient handling', *Giornale Italiano di Medicina del Lavoro* 90 (2): 399–411.

Personick, M.E. (1990) 'Nursing home aides experience increase in serious injuries', *Monthly Labour Review* 113 (2): 30–7.

Pilling, S. (1993) 'Calculating the risk', *Nursing Standard* 8 (6): 18–20.

Poll, K.J. (1987) 'Patient lifting, an ergonomic approach', *Musculoskeletal Disorders at Work*, London: Taylor & Francis, 247–9.

Prezant, B., Demers, P. and Strand, K. (1987) 'Back problems, training experience, and use of lifting aids among hospital nurses', in Asfour, S. (ed.) *Trends in Ergonomics/Human Factors IV*, Holland: Elsevier Science Publishers B.V., 839–45.

Raine, E. (2001) 'Testing a risk assessment tool for manual handling', *Professional Nurse* 16 (9): 1344–8.

Retsas, A. and Pinikahana, J. (1999) 'Manual handling practices and injuries among ICU nurses', *Australian Journal of Advanced Nursing* 17 (1): 37–42.

Retsas, A. and Pinikahana, J. (2000) 'Manual handling activities and injuries among nurses: an Australian hospital study', *Journal of Advanced Nursing* 31 (4): 875–83.

Ricci, M.G., Menoni, O., Colombini, D. and Occhipinti, E. (1999) 'Clinical studies in health workers employed in the manual lifting of patients: methods for the examination of spinal lesions', *Giornale Italiano di Medicina del Lavoro* 90: 173–90.

Rice, V.E. (1986) 'Low back pain among community nurses', *Journal of Occupational Health & Safety – Australia & New Zealand* 2: 134–7.

Rockefeller, K., Silverstein, B. and Howard, N. (2000) 'Getting to zero-lift in Washington state nursing homes', *Proceedings of the IEA2000/HFES 2000 Congress,* The Human Factors and Ergonomics Society, California: Santa Monica, 430–3.

Ryden, L.A., Molgaard, C.A., Bobbitt, S. and Conway, J. (1989) 'Occupational low-back injury in a hospital employee population: an epidemiologic analysis of multiple risk factors of a high-risk occupational group', *Spine* 14 (4): 315–30.

Rylands, J.M., Pike, I., Allan, L., Koehoorn, M., Mitchell, J. and Davison, D. (1994) 'A multi-level approach to ergonomic and related issues in the BC healthcare industry', in Robertson, S. (ed.) *Contemporary Ergonomics. Proceedings of the Ergonomics Society Annual Conference,* 434–9.

Scholey, M. and Hair, M.D. (1989) 'The problem of back pain in physiotherapists', *Physiotherapy Practice* 5: 183–92.

Scholey, M. and Hair, M. (1989) 'Back pain in physiotherapists involved in back care education', *Ergonomics* 32 (2): 179–90.

Shigeta, S., Misawa, T., Aikawa, H. and Kondo, A. (1979) 'An experimental study of nursing work load on the low back, *Japanese Journal of Industrial Health* 21: 164–70.

Skewes, S.M. (1997) 'Bathing: it's a tough job', *Journal of Gerontological Nursing* 45–9.

Smedley, J., Egger, P., Cooper, C. and Coggon, D. (1997) 'Prospective cohort study of predictors of incident low back pain in nurses', *British Medical Journal* 314: 1225–8.

Smedley, J., Inskip, H., Cooper, C. and Coggon, D. (1998) 'Natural history of low back pain. A longitudinal study in nurses', *Spine* 23: 2422–6.

Smith, N. (1996) 'Progression towards a "no manual lifting policy" within the intensive care unit', *Nursing in Critical Care* 1 (5): 237–40.

Sondergaard, T. (1976) 'Who considers the back of hospital personnel? Manual lifting saves minutes but one does not think of the sequelae', *Sygeplejersken* 76: 18–19.

St Vincent, M., Tellier, C. and Petitjean-Roget, T. (1999) 'Accidents that occurred in three hospitals in one year', *Safety Science* 31: 197–212.

Stacey, N. (1994) 'Benefits of moving and handling equipment', *British Journal of Therapy and Rehabilitation* 1 (1): 26–33.

Stobbe, T.J., Plummer, R.W., Jensen, R.C. and Attfield, M.D. (1988) 'Incidence of low back injuries among nursing personnel as a function of patient lifting frequency', *Journal of Safety Research* 19: 21–8.

Stubbs, D.A., Buckle, P., Hudson, M.P., Rivers, P.M. and Worringham, C.J. (1983) 'Back pain in the nursing profession: 1. epidemiology and pilot methodology', *Ergonomics* 26 (8): 755–65.

Torgén, M., Nygård, C. and Kilbom, A. (1995) 'Physical work load, physical capacity and strain among elderly female aides in home-care service', *European Journal of Applied Physiology* 71: 444–52.

Tracey, C. (1997) 'To lift or not to lift: 1. the legal requirements for patient lifting', *British Journal of Therapy and Rehabilitation* 4 (5): 234–9.

Tracey, C. (1997) 'To lift or not to lift: 2. the implications for patient lifting', *British Journal of Therapy and Rehabilitation* 4 (6): 332–9.

Triolo, P.K. (1989) 'Occupational health hazards for hospital staff nurses', *AAOHN Journal* 37 (7): 274–9.

Troup, J.D.G. (1982) 'Training in the handling of patients: the demands on education and occupational health for nurses', *Nurse Education Today* 2 (2): 13–15.

Turnbull, N., Dornan, J., Fletcher, B. and Wilson, S. (1992) 'Prevalence of spinal pain among the staff of a district health authority', *Occupational Medicine*, 143–8.

Uber, D., Foradori, M. and Cognola, M. (1999) 'Preliminary data on shoulder disorders in workers exposed to risk due to patient lifting in geriatric residences in the province of Trento', *Giornale Italiano di Medicina del Lavoro* 90: 350.

Uhl, J.E., Wilkinson, W.E. and Wilkinson, C.S. (1987) 'Aching backs? A glimpse into the hazards of nursing', *AAOHN Journal* 35 (1): 13–17.

Vasiliadou, A., Karvountzis, G., Roumeliotis, D., Soumilas, A., Plati, C. and Nomikos, I. (1997) 'Factors associated with back pain in nursing staff: a survey in Athens, Greece', *International Journal of Nursing Practice* 3: 15–20.

Vasiliadou, A., Karvountzis, G.G., Soumilas, A., Roumeliotis, D. and Theodosopoulou, E. (1995) 'Occupational low-back pain in nursing staff in a Greek hospital', *Journal of Advanced Nursing* 21: 125–30.

Venning, P.J. (1988) 'Back injury prevention. Instructional design features for program planning', *AAOHN Journal* 36: 336–41.

Venning, P.J., Walter, S.D. and Stitt, L.W. (1987) 'Personal and job-related factors as determinants of incidence of back injuries among nursing personnel', *Journal of Occupational Medicine* 29 (10): 820–5.

Videman, T., Nurminen, T., Tola, S., Kuorinka, I., Vanharanta, H. and Troup, J.D. (1984) 'Low-back pain in nurses and some loading factors of work 9: 400–4.

Vojtecky, M.A., Harber, P., Sayre, J.W., Billet, E. and Shimozaki, S. (1987) 'The use of assistance while lifting', *Journal of Safety Research* 18: 49–56.

Ward, L. and Knappett, J. (1995) 'A study to discuss manual handling training for home care staff in the constituency of Keighley', in *Proceedings of the National Back Exchange Conference*, University of Nottingham.

Watt, S. (1987) 'Nurses back injury, reducing the strain', *The Australian Nurses Journal* 16 (6): 46–7.

Wihlidal, L.M. and Kumar, S. (1997) 'An injury profile of practicing diagnostic medical sonographers in Alberta', *International Journal of Industrial Ergonomics* 19: 205–16.

PROFESSIONAL OPINION

Allen, A. (1990) 'On-the-job injury: a costly problem', *Journal of Post Anaesthesia Nursing* 5: 367–8.

Allen, L., Thompson, E. and Donaldson, L. (1999) 'Risk assessment – lateral transfers', *The Column* 11 (2): 16–17.

Anon. (1972) 'Stop, think – then lift', *Nursing Mirror & Midwives Journal* June 23: 9–11.

Anon. (1972) 'Hospital training for ambulance men', *Royal Society of Health Journal* 92 (3): 103.

Anon. (1984) 'Back savers', *Nursing Times Community Outlook*, October 10: 362–6.

Anon. (1990) 'Equipment to save your back', *Nursing Standard* 4: 26–7.

Anon. (1995) 'Professional development. Lifting and handling: knowledge for practice (continuing education credit)', *Nursing Times* 91: (suppl–4).

Anon. (1995) 'Professional development. Lifting and handling: revision notes (continuing education credit)', *Nursing Times* 9 (3: suppl–12): 9–14.

Anon. (1997) 'Handle nurses with care', *Nursing Times* 93, 4.

Bannister, C. (1996) 'Learning not to lift', *Nursing Standard* 11 (2): 25–6.

Bannister, C. and Hodgson, J. (1991) 'Watch your back', *Nursing Standard* 5 (33): 50–1.

Barker, A.C. (1995) 'Equipment for moving and handling', *British Journal of Therapy and Rehabilitation* 2 (10): 525–31.

Bates, J. (1989) 'Queensland nursing homes & hostels manual handling project. A joint project to reduce back injuries', *Queensland Nurse* 8: 14–15.

Bell, A. (1975) 'Hospitals harbour hazards ignored in fight for life', *International Journal of Occupational Health & Safety* 44: 26–9.

Beresford, S.A. (1997) 'Bath lifts and hoists', *British Journal of Therapy and Rehabilitation* 4 (4): 171–8.

Blue, C.L. (1996) 'Preventing back injury among nurses', *Orthopaedic Nursing* 15 (6): 9–21.

Brewer, S. (1993) 'The back injury battle', *Nursing Standard* 7 (40): 20–1.

Carlisle, D. (1992) 'Lifting developments', *Nursing Times* 88 (44): 42–4.

Carlowe, J. (1998) 'Reducing risks in lifting and handling', *Nursing Times* 94 (18): 62–4.

Charlesworth, S. (2000) 'Moving and handling and challenging behaviour', *The Column*: 26–7.

Clements, S. (1990) 'Taking the strain', *Nursing the Elderly:* 12–13.

Cohen, P. (1998) 'Moving and handling in the community', *Nursing Times* 94 (5): 4–5.

Couzens-Howard, D. and Williams, M. (1993) 'Essential support', *Nursing Times* 89 (6): 44–6.

Davey, M. (1990) 'Making light of lifting', *The Australian Nurses Journal* 19 (8): 20–1.

Dixon, M. (1968) 'Heavy lifting: bogy of nursing', *Nursing Times* 64: 1755.

Dower, T. (1999) 'Lighten the load', *Collegian* 6 (suppl–3): 12–14.

Duffy, B.S.C. and Duffy, C.L. (1994) 'Positioning patients: a different angle', *Journal of Clinical* 3: 197–8.

Erikson, K. and Goldschmidt, A. (1979) 'Education and training will keep the back free of injury', *Sygeplejersken* 18: 12–14.

Farmer, P. (1987) 'Mechanical aids', *Nursing Times* 83: 36–7.

Fitzgerald, J. and McCarthy, M. (1986) 'Back pain: safe lifting techniques', *World of Irish Nursing* 15: 5–6.

Fosnaught, M. (1999) 'PTs at Risk', *PT Magazine,* April: 35–40.

Fragala, G. (1994) 'Using ergonomics to prevent back injuries', *Nursing Management (Chicago)* 25 (10): 98–100.

Fragala, G. and Shelton, F. (1998) 'Applying the concepts of ergonomics to improve healthcare bed design', *Rehab and Therapy Products Review,* May/June.

Fredericks, S. (1993) 'Caring for your back', *Nursing New Zealand* August, 1: 11.

Gallagher, S. (2000) 'Meeting the needs of the obese patient', *American Journal of Nursing* 3–14.

Garg, A. (1993) 'What basis exists for training workers in "correct" lifting technique?' in Marras, W.S., Karwowski, W., Smith, J.L. and Pacholski, L. (eds) *The Ergonomics of Manual Work: Proceedings of the IEA world conference, Poland 14–17 June*, London: Taylor & Francis, 89–91.

Gonet, L. and Kryzwon, A. (1991) 'Preventing back pain through education', *Nursing Standard* 5 (24): 25–7.

Griffin, V. (1987) 'Back injuries: 2. the stories behind the statistics', *Queensland Nurse* 6: 15–17.

Haley, E. (1994) 'One approach to patient lifting', *The Canadian Nurse,* 57–9.

Hancock, C. (1996) 'Risky business', *Nursing Standard* 10 (29): 16.

Harlev., J. (1992) 'Work environment – investing in good lifting technique', *Sygeplejersken* 92: 12–13.

Hayne, C. (1984) 'Safe patient movement – an alternative approach', *Medical Education (International) Ltd,* 931–65.

Hearn, V. (1988) 'Safe lifting and moving for nurse and patient', *Nursing – Oxford* 3: 9–12.

Helmlinger, C. (1997) 'A growing physical workload threatens nurses' health', *Issues Update* 97 (4).

Hocking, J. (1996) 'A back-breaking workload', *Nursing Times* 94 (46): 62–4.

Hogan, M. (1994) 'Heavier than normal handling – say no to back injuries', *Australian Nursing Journal* 1 (8): 14.

Hollis, M. (1992) 'A review of liability reports in healthcare environments', *Occupational Health*, 296–8.

Howie, C. (1982) 'Oh, my back', *Nursing Times* November 17: 1937–8.

Huck, L. (1996) 'Strategies for altering practice', *Nursing Times* 92 (15): 29–30.

Jannings, W. and Armitage, S. (1996) 'The community nursing environment: back care considerations', *Journal of Occupational Health & Safety – Australia & New Zealand* 12 (4): 423–9.

Jensen, L.K. and Hansen, H.B. (1986) 'Working environment. Many work impediments among personnel in operating room', *Sygeplejersken* 47: 4–10.

Lenihan, J. (1983) 'Design in health care. Problem of back injuries in nursing. Taking the strain', *Nursing Mirror*, June 29: 25–6.

Lloyd, P. (1986) 'Handle with care', *Nursing Times*, November 19, 82: 33–5.

Lloyd, P. (1987) 'Back pain in nurses', *Occupational Health* 39: 109–10.

Lloyd, P. (1989) 'Manual handling', *Occupational Health* 41: 22–3.

Lloyd, P. (1990) 'Handling techniques for nurses', *Nursing Standard* 4 (25): 24–5.

Lloyd, P.V. (1981) 'Back pain – prevention not cure', *Nursing Focus* 3: 460–1.

Love, C. (1993) 'Lifting patients: the challenge for nursing', *Nursing Standard* 7 (27): 27–9.

MacFarlane, E. (1995) 'Whose back is it?' *British Journal of Theatre Nursing*. 4 (11): 8–12.

Marchette, L. and Marchette, B. (1985) 'Back injury: a preventable occupational hazard', *Orthopaedic Nursing* 4: 25–9.

Mathias, J.M. (2000) 'Taking a load off OR personnel', *OR Manager* 16 (7): 12.

McCall, J. (1991) 'Watch your back', *Nursing Standard* 5 (24): 50–1.

Meadows, L. (2001) 'Therapeutic handling', *The Column*, August: 22–3.

Naish (1996) 'Campaign aims to change the culture on manual lifting', *Nursing Times* 20 (15): 27–30.

Nawar, M. (2000) 'Back me up: stop injuries now', *American Nurse* 32: 22–3.

Okunowo, R. (1992) 'Home truths', *Nursing Standard* 6 (32): 55.

Oliveck, M. (1998) 'Lifts and hoists', *Therapy Weekly* July 16: 6.

Østby, B.A. and Herdlevær, A.S. (1985) 'Danish study demonstrates: nursing personnel has record in back injuries', *Sykepleien* 72: 16–18.

Owen, B.D. (2000) 'Preventing injuries using an ergonomic approach', *AORN Journal* 72 (6): 1031–6.

Patterson, D. (1993) 'Minimizing back injuries in nursing home staff', *Nursing Homes*, Jan./Feb. 33–4.

Reed, A.G. (1982) 'Think back', *Nursing Focus* 3: 12–14.

Reed, M. (1983) 'Design in health care. Backing education', *Nursing Mirror*, June 29: 30.

Roche, N. (1999) 'Back injuries still common despite modern equipment', *The World of Irish Nursing*, June: 16–17.

Rogers, P. (1983) 'Sharing the load', *Nursing Mirror*, June 29: 28–9.

Ruszala, S. (1999) 'Selecting a hospital bed', *The Column* 11 (3): 12–16.

Sadler, C. (1991) 'BACKUP – Back injuries at work are preventable, and nurses can hold their employees responsible for implementing safe working practices', *Nursing Times* 87 (11): 16–17.

Schaeffer, J.N. and Millen, H. (1950) 'Controlling risks in patient transfers', *Hospitals* 54: 46.

Scholey, M. (1984) 'Patient handling skills', *Nursing Times*, June 27, 80: 24–7.

Schuldenfrei, P. (1998) 'No heavy lifting. Making safety work', *American Journal of Nursing* 98: 46–8.

Scott, K. (1999) 'Slide to safety', *The Column* 11 (4): 20–1.

Sedgley-Roach, T.S. (1992) 'Avoiding an unnecessary strain – an examination of listing practice', *Professional Nurse*: 453–6.

Seymour J. (1995) 'Lifting and moving patients', *Nursing Times* 91 (27): 48–50.

Shaw, R. (1981) 'Creating back care awareness', *Dimensions in Health Service* 58: 32–3.

Snell, J. (1998) 'Lifting the burden', *Health Service Journal,* 29 January: 8–9.

Sopher, B.J. (1994) 'Will manual handling regulations reduce the incidence of back disorders?' *Occupational Medicine* 44: 267.

Swiatczak, L. (1992) 'Lifting and moving', *Nursing the Elderly* 4 (5): 40–1.

Tarling, C. (1992) 'The right equipment', *Nursing Times* 88 (50): 38–40.

Tarling, C. and Burns, N. (1994) 'Let the bed take the strain: an ergonomic approach to hospital bed provision', *Professional Nurse,* 759–63.

Trascz, S. and Rose L. (1983) 'National study could help beat back injury', *Dimensions*: 22–3.

Vasey, J. and Crozier, L. (1982a) 'A move in the right direction', *Nursing Mirror*, April 28: 42–7.

Vasey, J. and Crozier, L. (1982b) 'At ease', *Nursing Mirror*, May 12: 28–31.

Vasey, J. and Crozier, L. (1982c) 'Easy on the base', *Nursing Mirror*, May 26: 36–42.

Vasey, J. and Crozier, L (1982d) 'Get in condition', *Nursing Mirror*, May 5: 22–8.

Vasey, J. and Crozier, L. (1982e) 'Handle with care', *Nursing Mirror*, May 19: 30–2.

Vasey, J. and Crozier, L. (1982f) 'Safety first', *Nursing Mirror*, June 2: 44–8.

Vousden, M. (1989) 'A pain in the back', *Nursing Times* 85 (3): 19.

Walsh, R. (1988) 'Good movement habits', *Nursing Times* 84 (37): 49–61.

Waters, J. (1997) 'Reducing the risks from lifting', *Nursing Times* 93 (50): 52–4.

Waters, J. (1998) 'Hidden hazards associated with moving and handling', *Community Nurse* 4: 21–2.

Westbrook, S. (1995) 'Donway traction splint', *Accident & Emergency Nursing* 3: 226–7.

White, C. (1998) 'Back breaking work', *Nursing Times* 94 (40): 24–6.

White, C. (1999) 'Backs at work', *Nursing Times* 95 (5): 57–9.

White, C. (1999) 'Preventing injuries at work', *Nursing Times* 95 (34): 54–8.

Willer, S. (1989) 'A new approach to back injury', *Nursing Standard* 46 (3): 32–3.

Williams, K. (1996) 'Handle with care', *Nursing Standard* 10 (28): 26–7.

Williams, L. and Coleman, S. (1999) 'Patient hoist sling evaluation', (1998) *The Column* 11 (2): 15–16.

Wilson, M. (1986) 'Lifting patients: mind your backs', *Community Outlook*: 11–14.

Wilson, M., Forbes, R. and Mitchell, L. (1998) 'Do your nurses get injured lifting clients? If they do – you should read this!' *JARNA* 1 (4): 7–8.

Woodcraft, B. (1991) 'Uplifting experience?' *Nursing Standard* 6 (6): 55–6.

Wright, B. (1992) 'Patient handling – let's get it right', *Nursing Standard* 6: 52–3.

NOT PRIMARY SOURCE

Baty, D., Stubbs, D.A., Buckle, P.Q., Hudson, M.P. and Rivers, P.M. (1985) 'Working postures and associated stress in a nursing population', in Brown, I. *et al.* (eds) *Ergonomics International 85, Proceedings of the 9th Congress of IEA*, Paris: The International Ergonomics Association, 463–5.

Charney, W. (1992) 'The lifting team: second year data reported [news]', *AAOHN Journal* 40: 503.

Collins, J.W. and Owen B. (1996) 'NIOSH research initiatives to prevent back injuries to nursing assistants, aides, and orderlies in nursing homes', *American Journal of Industrial Medicine* 29: 421–4.

Engkvist, I.L., Wigaeus-Hjelm, E. and Hagberg, M. (2000) 'Patient transfers and the preventative effects for over-exertion back injury of training and use of transfer devices among nursing personnel', *Proceedings of the IEA2000/HFES 2000 Congress*, The Human Factors and Ergonomics Association, California: Santa Monica, 5: 427–9.

Feldstein, A., Vollmer, W. and Valanis, B. (1990) 'Evaluating the patient-handling tasks of nurses', *Journal of Occupational Medicine* 32 (10): 1009–13.

Garg, A. and Owen, B. (1991) 'A biomechanical and ergonomic evaluation of patient transferring tasks', in Queinnec, Y. and Daniellou, F. (eds) *Designing for Everyone, Proceedings of the 11th congress of the IEA, Paris*, London: Taylor & Francis 1: 60–2.

Hignett, S. (1996) 'Midwifery – managing the manual handling risks', in Robertson, S. (ed.) *Contemporary Ergonomics. Proceedings of the Ergonomics Society annual conference*, London: Taylor & Francis, 415–20.

Hignett, S. (1999) 'Hands-on approach', *Occupational Health* 51: 23–5.

Hignett, S. (2000) 'Reducing risks in occupational therapy practice', *Proceedings of the IEA2000/HFES 2000 Congress*, The Human Factors and Ergonomics Society, California: Santa Monica, 4: 272.

Jensen, R. (1990) 'Prevention of back injuries among nursing staff', in Charney, W. and Schirmer, J. *Essentials of Modern Hospital Safety (*Chapter 14), Lewis Publishers, 237–57.

Lagerström, M., Josephson, M., Pingel, B., Tjernström, G. and Hagberg, M. (1998) 'Evaluation of the implementation of an education and training programme for nursing personnel at a hospital in Sweden', *International Journal of Industrial Ergonomics* 21: 79–90.

Marras, W.S., Davis, K.G., Kirking, B.C. and Bertsche, P.K. (1998) 'Low back disorder and spinal load during patient transfer', *Proceedings of the IEA 1998/HFES 1998 Congress*, London: Taylor & Francis, 901–5.

Owen, B. and Garg, A. (1991) 'Approaches to reducing back stress for nursing personnel', in Karwowski, W. and Yates, J.W. (eds) *Advances in Industrial Ergonomics and Safety III* London: Taylor & Francis, 513–20.

Owen, B.D. and Garg, A. (1991) 'A reducing risk for back pain in nursing personnel', *AAOHN Journal* 39: 24–33.

Owen, B.D. and Garg, A. (1993) 'Back stress isn't part of the job', *American Journal of Nursing* 93: 48–51.

St Vincent, M., Lortie, M. and Tellier, C. (1987) 'A new approach for the evaluation of training programs in safe lifting', in Asfour, S. (ed.) *Trends in Ergonomics/Human Factors IV*, Holland, Elsevier Science Publishers B.V., 847–55.

Trevelyan, F. (2001) 'The implementation and evaluation of an ergonomics intervention in an acute hospital', *The Column* 13 (1): 22–4.

Trevelyan, F. and Buckle, P. (2000) 'Change in exposure to risk for back pain following an ergonomics intervention in an acute hospital', *Proceedings of the IEA2000/HFES 2000 Congress*, The Human Factors and Ergonomics Society, California, Santa Monica, 5: 423–6.

Wachs, J.E. and Parker-Conrad, J.E. (1989) 'Predictors of registered nurses' lifting behaviour', *AOHN Journal* 37 (4): 131–40.

INDEX